The Humble Schizophrenic

A Poem in Introduction

I hear voices.

Hello, is there anybody out tl
My name is Pete.
Things were groovy once,
Things were dire at another time
Now they are the same.
Where did it start?
What rotten stinker did it?
Well I will tell you where it started,
There I was playing Shostakovich's string quartet, number 3
Like I was doing because I needed a groove
And some guy, some guy I did not know says through the wall -
"You play guitar well."
Well if I could talk through the wall at that exact time that is exactly what I would have said.
But the question had to arise
How the fuck did you talk through the wall
But I was brought up to have manners so I said thanks
Through the wall back to him.

Where was the wall
It was across the wall
It was in front yet from behind me
A new dawn had approached, presenting itself.
A new dawn of telepathic hoodoo.

A month of this and I had left.
Ejits introducing themselves
Bastards outside saying they'd make me talk when I was
Quiet
Having long hood wink chats before I went to bed
No television my dad had said, you won't study
Surrounded by people taking a break
The spiritualist government
The national infra structure of the mind
I don't dig it I don't need it I only hear it and
Talk
When I felt like it and that was a lot of the hours

Minutes went by and it was time to leave
Blood dripping from my wrist
Pull out of everything necessary
Take away everything I was pushing
Time to go on a calling, a change
A career and this is a story in which I may appear.

The Humble Schizophrenic

Pete's Escape

brentpower@gmail.com

Peter

Peter Brown

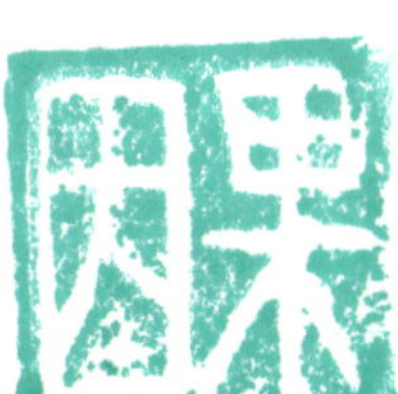

chipmunkapublishing
the mental health publisher

Published by
Chipmunkapublishing
PO Box 6872
Brentwood
Essex CM13 1ZT
United Kingdom

http://www.chipmunkapublishing.com

Edited by Aleks Lech

Chipmunkapublishing gratefully acknowledge the support of Arts Council England.

God looked down…they knew Pete.

God looked down upon Voodoo man, a twenty year old who often stared up at God, searching for some father figure that he had lost long ago. God would have smiled down on him, he would then have inhaled God's spirit, then turn away, promptly denying to himself where that momentary love had come from, and march onwards, sore.

Recently though he had let himself drift further away from God (who always looked down) and had grown somewhat annoyed and resentful of God, the God he could less and less look in the eye. And so he had begun to manipulate his associates and friends. The darkness this entailed had begun to drive his life. He was getting more and more out of control. This change was influencing his mind but he wondered,

"It was just the end of puberty or something. After all the world allows it." He was giddy as his new life spun around his thoughts.

It was in this sensitive state he bumped into Pete.

God looked down on Joe Bob. Joe Bob, an angelic refugee, had made a mistake around the fall of his then friend - the devil (from the grace of God). God felt the best way for him to learn and mend his ways was to live with the humans polluted by sin from Eden. He was filtered down generation by generation, as some new family's son. They say "God works in mysterious ways". That "God is benevolent." No such way was evidently more "mysterious" or "benevolent" than the fact that God wiped Joe Bob's memory clean with each incarnation and new family. God would alert each set of parents to his identity by a visitation, just as the virgin Mary had been told about Jesus' birth. Secret historians had documented all of his lives in secret books. These historians were alerted to his lives as this peculiar arrangement implemented by God always caused curiosity from the hidden world of spirits, a place that withheld few secrets.

Although blind to the results and lessons of each of his five hundred odd lives he was beginning to learn how to beat these historians, parents and others by a second nature that could not be denied to him. Recent lives had been an extravagant cat and mouse game with them. He denied them their victories and his actions were more and more often leaving them confused and baffled. He was likened to a "skilled swordsman who was blind." He remembered life mistakes like distant uncertain dreams.

Yet unbeknown to him he would meet a good friend in this life – Pete, who would confirm to him the lives he suspected he had lived, have a final victory and a reconciliation.

God looked down on Wolfie. Wolfie was dead. God disliked looking at the dead for a good reason. The dead were always aware of His sight, any influences that would have leaked into their subconsciousness they would have been unaware of when they had been living where now noticed. Now if they saw God looking down on them they would rejoice for days, thinking he was praising them and then thinking they were righteous - a massive false exaltation. They would try and teach disciples. It would evidently all cause harm.

God left the dead alone but some people could see God. People who had witnessed His spirit during their lifetime, they knew God saw them, and they did not bother Him. They waited for His return.

Where was Wolfie in this relationship? During life he had been a successful businessman. God had just looked down on him and he was reminded of a strange feeling, a feeling he had shunned during his life many times. He immediately knew who it had come from; in shame he did not look up. He appeared in front of Pete. He acknowledged a sallow thin young man with straw hair in some distress. And there he was, but he was silent for now.

God looked down on Nile. Nile was a collective of demonic forces, Nile were immediately aware of what had happened and did not need to look or meet His eyes to know whose gaze rested on them.

"Fuck off!" they snarled to God. They were aggressive to God, but the less they saw him the better, as this momentary engagement with Righteousness had killed off a section of them. They swarmed away spinning and cutting, sucked in a metaphysical vacuum which formed as they had nothing to engage or hurt. For now they could not think, they fell infinite metres banging off sharp rocks. They spread, cursing one another but from far off they saw a light. They soared to it.

They seemed to have arrived in some sort of hospital. They searched for whom they might devour. Pete was there relaxed on a bed, reading.

God looked down on Imooman. A human who was many millions of light years from his native earth, the same earth the readers call home. Imoonan had the fine facial features and ebony skin of a south American Indian. God watched him operating his spaceship and He followed the electric currents travelling through a multitude of crude circuit boards, centuries old. This old ship was cumbersome but technologically advanced for the period of time it came from. It had been made during the classical period of his race's existence (around 680 AD). Any documents that described the times and how the ship had been forged had been destroyed by the old Indian priests.

They did this because they felt the invading Spanish and their conquistadors were just not ready for such knowledge. They had been right. The priests had tried to help the Europeans by simple directions they had left in scrolls, but these were seen as the devil's work and destroyed. It was ironic, Imoonan thought, that many of the governments would do anything for the knowledge that ancestors had destroyed.

This strange sight did not overwhelm God, he just saw a lonely man around thirty years of age. God decided he would point Imoonan back to earth.

"I think I will go back to earth" Imoonan pondered, so he went against the distaste he had for present day civilisation, he twitched a computer's dials on a gold dash, he heard the buzz of the many thousands of its intricate cogs. Archaic symbols clicked into place in front of him. There was a possible route, he needed to do some business anyway, why else would he go? After all he never picked up any consumer culture morons who could not shirk and even liked the massive control they were under by "the powers." Old prophesies had foreseen one would change all this but he could not see this happening in his age.

God looked down on Jackie. Jackie was newly married and had become a house wife, though did work part time. Also she was trying at becoming a medium. She thought about her friend who had introduced her to the Spiritualist Church. She would have plenty of time to talk to the dead, God chuckled.

She sat at the table as her husband did the dishes, happily thinking. How lucky, how contented she was. She talked about some old cow she knew at work. There was a certain ominous entity keeping its distance, watching. She thought to next Wednesday and noticed it. Spiritualist night was on Wednesday and she mistook the entity for some future challenge.

Though God loved her and with one tiny thought He ruined the future and destiny that the church elders and "higher beings" had planned for Jackie. He would provide her with a more noble quest, one he would involve Pete in too. It would dwarf what any that these "other elders" and church spirits could imagine.

God looked down on Kelsang. He watched an Asian man dressed in orange robes. He concentrated on the man and said,

"Stupid monk." Then "Ah Kelsang."

God mulled over this. The man did not hear, he just walked. He had been journeying for many months by way of many countries, mostly foreign to his spiritual identity. Yet God had caused this exodus, this leaving from his familiar world. The monk had escaped from a country where he and his friends had been persecuted. He had found a Buddhist temple in the far away land he had just entered. He told its Abbot about his travels and needs;

"Where is the most forsaken city in this continent?"

"Ah," the Abbot said, "It is City 29."

God smiled; Pete lived there.

Chapter 1
The straight doctor

A stupid scribble on the wall, a wall of charts and his certificates, both of which the doctor was immensely proud of.

"Done by his child." thought Pete.

"Let's bring it up for a laugh." Pete spoke to himself.

"Do you believe in ritual magic?" Bang, there it was. Pete had sort of watched these words flow from his mouth...

" Ritual magic? What's that?" The doctor slouched in his business swivel chair. He was focusing his mind by folding his hands together in a gesture of complete understanding that left behind his honest body language, which would have been one of ridicule. This technique was one learnt by a conditioning of sorts. An honest relationship on his side would not expose this boy's neurosis and so one enticed. It began with a trickle;

"You know voodoo. It troubles me. It promotes a parallel world to the physical world in every respect. There is harm in an exchange through body to body as there is harm exchanged from the mind to a mind."

"Whose mind?" he asked, with intent to challenge his reasoning; perhaps somewhere in his subconscious he was interested but he had a job to do.

"Well," Pete said replying as the doc had asked. He stopped. He wondered did the shrink really wanted to know?

"Why not?" Pete reflected in a logical way.

"It is using compassion to know such knowledge, a knowledge that can facilitate the creation of further acts of infinite compassion. Am I bad? People think I am odd."

He'd said it aloud; there it was, that was Pete's enlightenment. He mumbled,

"....for me it is everybody, at least everybody or even everything."

The Doctor was no longer listening; he was scribbling away on his records with a golden tipped fountain pen. Pete began to rationalise.

" I only position myself in a place I find amicable in life, one where I can be compassionate, that isn't ritual magic it's only common sense. I mean by magic trying to influence the power of prayer. Who alive cares about your actions anyway? Everyone's too busy with their own. So this way isn't fraught with much difficulty, when you decide to desert your place in some universal mindscape, (the doctor looked up) and become a devotee of this compassion, negative energy chases you, asking you to pay, pay for all his, ah "evil" is the only word I can think of. It's a crazy life; I like it."

The doctor hadn't spoke for several minutes. That last statement prompted him to reason;

"He has a messiah complex."

This thought then morphed into connecting Pete's confession with schizoid tendencies, possibly underpinned by some depletion of the serotonin levels in the brain. Using his psychiatric training he decided to pretend he was perplexed. Pete had stopped talking. The doctor was smiling, Pete was looking out of the window glad of the country's mild climate; it was the end of winter, the birds would be on their return migration.

"An uneventful journey home." he dreamed, picturing it.

He got up, expecting the doctor to mutter "another three months" and so pushed the seat backwards and said,

"Good bye."

Raising his hand to signal Pete to hold on the doctor made a phone call. Pete was used to this rudeness but as the call finished an orderly in a white coat appeared at the door.

Chapter 2
Thank God Lobotomies are Defunct

They hauled Pete's ass down avenues of sparsely decorated rooms full of those who perceived themselves wrongly confined, the doctor's inmates. It was all too much, no nice bus ride home.

"I was going to have soup for lunch." Pete almost cried.

Pete was pushed into a large room. There was a cupboard full of pharmaceutical dictionaries and other rarely read books which were on policy and psychiatric protocols. At the front of this room's window the orderly called Mickey pulled out a seat and another tall man put his hands on Pete's shoulders in a sort of motion that told him to sit down right there.

"Hi there, my name is Mickey. I am the senior charge nurse here in Meadowbank hospital. You are being detained under the Mental Health Act of 1986. You will be put under observation; everything is here." A nurse handed Pete a document of several pages. It was read and basically said firstly that they could forcibly medicate him and secondly the section would be reviewed in 14 days and lastly that they could give him ECT - electric shock therapy!

"You sign at the bottom." Micky said, in his helpful nurse speak.

"Go fuck yourself." Pete said.

Sometimes when you have to look after yourself there is no room for compassion.

They dragged him by his arms and forcibly ejected him into one of the rooms that had beds in them (this one had a double of the auxiliary nurse sitting outside it). They walked back leaving Pete, not turning round; one more delinquent. They left to leave him to slowly give the room the once over.

A wardrobe, a bed, a desk and seat and a window that looked out into the bottom of a hill. (When the ward was built it had been carefully landscaped). There was also an en suite shower room and toilet.

Pete with a lot of might returned himself to his usual demeanour of charity and said

"Well, I will make the most of my time here."

And Pete lay back on the bed thinking he might ponder the mysteries of the world now he had time.

"After all I have time."

He cried. Perhaps now he thought he might wake up and then he would be returned to his simple plans.

At this moment the ghost spirit Wolfie was passing by. He remembered this area 50 years ago as the same desolate place, now the large island of hospital wards surrounded by a motorway and some high rise flats. There were about sixteen buildings with lots of grass and as it was the winter - leafless trees. He noticed some of the buildings were new and had been built around the time of his death, though the others were eerie Victorian red brick ones that had housed patients for decades and still did. What about this new one he appeared in?

"This is strange."

Moments before he had just seen the eyes of God.

He stood in the Stevens Ward. He saw a trio of nurses at the bottom of a long corridor and, using his preferred method of travelling, he looked where they stood and there he was sliding towards them and controlling his speed like sideways gravity. No matter how many times he did this it still made him chuckle. He had slid too close; he was in the nurses' space, he fell back a couple of yards.

Chapter 3
A Busy Place

All that was there was a scrawny looking boy pondering and whispering to himself on a bed. Wolfie looked at him; the boy's actions on a second look were flowing through his world, picking virtual elements that could be found there, leaving other things and reverberating them back, changing them. Strange day dreams.

"He's called Pete" a dead relative called from the next room, causing Pete to reply,

"Yes I am" with a politeness that surprised the relative.

"What's he thinking?" uttered Wolfie. To his surprise the boy Pete blurted out a in a low witter that was also a substantiated reply;

"Accents man, more accurately they are lessons of a region. The way it works is people of a region stick to one lesson. When people speak to each other they identify with their speech as being something everyone knows, sort of unique individual lessons that vary from place to place. The lessons produce characteristics; they are class in the south, they dedicate themselves when talking to embellishing the positives of being class while being conscious of the negatives of being class, you know what I mean man? It‘s my singularity theory, the one thing included or left out illuminates everything, the whole language, it's in nature, time and time…"

"All I know," Wolfie blurted out, then thought about it, thought about his own voice,

"is well, I am a careful sort of guy."

"Let me demonstrate my theory. It works on individuals as well as collectives; you let yourself be dominated by this carefulness in return for being sure of your conduct! That is you all over. Though your accent is also carrying a regional lesson. Look, the Chinese speak in sounds, yet in Chinese there is no word for sound, this leads to lingual expression, leaving one and expressing the rest in it. It's all from history - confound the language that they may not understand one another's speech, Genesis 11. Before this was a mother tongue, a strange one without regions where the lesson they left out was their collective origin."

"Why are you here? I guess your thinking is bloody weird to surreal but why are you here, why are you talking to me?" Unexpectedly as he, Wolfie, spoke, the boy was uttering what he was saying out of his adam's apple. It was a way Pete had developed to listen with more attention.

"That's quaint" Wolfie thought.

But the boy didn't say "that's quaint" as Wolfie meant to keep it to himself. He looked back.

Wolfie muttered into the next room to the spirit that had made the previous introduction,

"He doesn't always hear me."

The patient in the next room yelped,

"I do, do."

This person's relative instructed Wolfie to go away as she was trying her best to calm her living kin who was suffering from some sort of mania. Wolfie was puzzled.

The boy he was looking at must have been excommunicated from normal society, that's why he was in this place;

"…he's conscious of my thoughts. He's a wreck, he's broken his programming. The alive are conditioned to being courteous to the dead, they are engaged in things they can only see in front of them, when they hear us they incorporate our words into an action, and if you want a living being to go against what's good you better have a good reason. That was it. No wonder he's here. Why has he done such a thing? He is broken, such an irreversible act, a person without destiny, he considered. But it was rare, there were noticeable personalities who had emerged, but..." Wolfie retreated into his own thoughts but kept an eye on this Pete.

He had been present at a go-between circle in some secret place, a designed place designated for the mortal and the dead, meant for camaraderie, though very tricky. Very controlled, heavily chaperoned. This was the only time before he had any such near direct contact with the living. It had caused him great worry. He had approached them, they all had looks and expressions of concentration but Wolfie couldn't connect, he'd retreated but the people had brought him back.

"I can't leave." he sobbed.

Suddenly a main spirit familiar with all this business raised a finger at him, and said,

"Be still" and he disappeared Wolfie did not like this way. An old woman with a maroon woollen pullover spoke; "I see…." She described Wolfie and said, "Please identify yourself, make yourself known. What is your business at our circle?" Wolfie could not leave so said his name and how he had arrived;

"I was at the church next door and I saw the front door was open, but I couldn't detect anyone and I came in and there you all were."

"He wishes us well." said the woman.

Wolfie hung out there for a bit and watched. Spirits in the room would disappear and one of the members would speak. The only worthwhile thing he saw take place was when a woman whose name was Jackie showed a great deal of compassion to a person who was experiencing a kind of reverse bereavement and she said that they would share love again. The head of the circle then glanced over at her and said to Jackie,

"Right, we will move on now."

The rest of the night Wolfie witnessed some gate-crashing and giggling. The official circle guides tried to reassert themselves and promote the idea that all people were to become responsible souls who would join together in the afterlife someday, and this seemed to be accepted except for the girl Jackie; her mind seemed a little bit awkward.

She secretly doubted.

Chapter 4
Becoming Friends

Back at Meadowbank the first day seemed to have worn Pete out. Wolfie reflected with an intuitive anticipation and said, "Pete is the guy that could teach that circle a few things! I will hang out with him for a few days and try help him out of here, but Pete and society as I know it; together, I dunno."

Pete drifted deeper and deeper into slumber, it was still twilight, dusk and a moonless night. The dark crept through the window over Pete's bed where outside a couple of psychiatric nurses (both thinking of what better things they could be doing) sat in the lit corridors of the ward, but Pete wasn't thinking that, he couldn't give a fuck.

Pete was now oblivious to his situation as he had entered the latter stages of r.e.m. sleep. Wolfie gazed at him, then the sleeping body looked back at him,

"Who are you?" it said.

"I am Wolfie, I want to be your friend."

Seeing the ghost like this confused Pete in his slumber and he told the ghost,

"I thought you were dead, but you appear in front of me."

Wolfie had had this happen before. It could help bereavement to appear in people's dreams, showing yourself in a dream to your dear one to show you were there and comforting when in hindsight. Though this case was different; when Pete woke up he would know what had happened, but that wouldn't concern or bother either of them. He slyly replied he wasn't dead, he didn't want him to give him any sort of jolt. Both liked each other and out of the nurses' earshot Pete was relaxed. He said that things had been groovy once, then he'd had the tripe beat out of his mind by someone; he had got away in the end, and now was in a more amicable situation.

Pete began to toss and turn, and continued,

"I am just chilling now, taking it easy. Getting away has shown me life is a wide expanse but I am not interested in it. Jesus has saved me, I am redeemed, he gave me a free ticket through life. Not only do I screw the usual life routes, but if I feel like it I go up to it and tell it to its face that I hate it or like it. And if I like it I will live it and when I am bored, well I will screw it. The ghosts don't always dig this though. Wait, ghosts? You are that guy…" and Pete sat up in bed and stopped the sleeping rant. He searched for Wolfie who was leaving the ward and said, "It's all right."

The next day two auxiliary nurses marched Pete with Wolfie in tow down to the dining hall. The two hands sat down with the other nurses at the door and Pete got sorted out with a hot chocolate and a scone. Looking around he didn't know any of the inmates.

"Or should he say patients?" There was a guy looking straight at him. Parts of his head were shaved and the bald spots had scars on them. Pete pondered and, sipping his hot chocolate but not forgetting this painful looking injury, he mulled it over; suddenly Pete had a black out, a shock of panic hit him, on the tail of which he heard, "He's had electro shocks, now fuck off!" It took a moment for Pete to realise he'd been shouted at by some touchy relative.

Angrily he shouted after them,

"I was only looking."

He looked away, and looked at three other inmates, they were jabbering about whether to play pool or contract whist. Pete would have to go back to his room, him being under observation with that mental health act. There were about fifteen to twenty patients and another six nurses in the dining hall. Two of the nurses were woman. They all had name tags, the two that were Pete's orderlies weren't real nurses, they were only hired hands, although all of them wore white shirts embroidered with the health trust logo (the organization that ran the hospital). There were real qualified nurses like Mickey who dished out the meds. But he was not there, he was away writing notes outlining 'progress.'

Back in Pete's assigned room it was getting late. An uneventful day. The nurses never slept during shifts, they had rotas; these guys were in for the whole night. Pete let Wolfie's voice come through him in a whisper, quiet so only he could hear it.

It was noticed within the dead's kingdom that Pete seemed to talk to anyone, he never backed off or shirked from any of their situations. Wolfie couldn't understand why Pete just didn't look away from the dead that approached him.

"Look away" he said. An adolescent who had been in this kingdom for many months and who felt he had got to grips with the extended protocol of continued existence was seeing if Pete, this mortal man, was up for partying like most of the dead peers he met.

"Nice to see ya" he said.

"Yeah man" Pete said. He gave the boy a smile.

This visitor paused, he felt a great deal of woe; seeing Pete lie there with all his awareness and his foresight of things he had only learned when born into death. To him Pete looked dead as he could see and wasn't "deaf" as people who had no sixth sense and were still in the mortal body were described. He felt sad and torn apart at Pete's existence.

"Look where he is." He looked much like himself except he lay there, not being able to get away, just looking at seemingly zilch.

Pete let his tongue dive into the spiritual realm in a bidding whisper to somewhere where he imagined there was someone who would help the ghost. No one came and he heaved a sigh.

"Oh well, c'est la vie."

There was one person who heard it but he wasn't the intended recipient, actually he was probably the least equipped to help Pete. The only reason he was drawn near to it was that he was offended that no one ever asked him for things like this. He was extremely foolish and resented the fact he had wasted his life both alive and dead. That's why he heard it; he was saying,

"Nobody ever asks me for jack shit" and there it was as usual flying past him. He stopped everything and watched.

"Why don't you get up, numbskull?"

Wolfie once again witnessed Pete talk to anyone and this time to a complete sociopath.

Pete replied he was perfectly content and just lying there, and that he was chilling with his friend Wolfie.

"Look at yourself, you should be out living, us dead are here to support you, you should stop your ghoulish pursuits, turn us off and make us just a memory or live with us properly devote yourself to a lifetime of substance, come on man…" He felt he was on to something here, he knew he could do it. Then Pete mumbled,

"Fucking naff off, I am happy I am not going to do any of your shit." Then Wolfie said,

"You should have listened to me, it's always better to ignore the likes of those two" This other ghost departed with his tail between his legs uttering "You'll get yours, just wait and you'll see."

Pete was not bothered.

Chapter 5
Enter the Unwelcome

As the jealous ghost huffed and cursed he was recognized. Someone was looking for hope, to turn hope to negativity, malice and disaster. Often these evil ones were witnessed doing their dastardly business. Yes, he'd seen this sort before, you could say, he had learnt to be an apologist to such goings on and he did not have the balls nor the guile to successfully translate just wishes to reality. He was pounced on. He was meeting Nile.

"Simple enough tell old Nile here your troubles."

"Well it's this jerk." He paused. He'd wanted to help that wretched boy, but this guy was all about pain.

"Come on, we could help." Fumbling about for words he hesitated and looked at his feet and in a moment he was falling. He had got himself into trouble and he could not handle it.

"Come on, tell." His legs were falling and he was burning, he could not see he could only feel Nile who he could feel was stoic and relaxed, electric with hate.

He looked at Nile and as the words came out he found himself on his own two feet back in the ward, his mood agreeable, but he'd spilled the beans on the boy. Nile was away but he was terrified, he knew one bad thought about this demon Nile and he'd be back. He sat and wondered about evil and devils. He had not done anything bad, he'd only introduced Pete. He was not going to do harm, he had not hurt Pete.

During this Pete was fast asleep. His door was propped open. The nurses sat outside; all of their small talk and conversation used up over hundreds of nights of doing the same work. Only the pay was good. Pete's neighbour though was sat up with the lights turned on. Delusions had robbed him of any sociability and his 'relative' wasn't around so he giggled at the nurses who'd whacked a downer into him, thinking he was fucking with them. He could hear snores from the next room, funny how your own snores don't wake you up he thought. Although everything was normal in Meadowbank an unnerving wind had started outside.

Pete dreamt. He saw a plague of flies, a sandstorm of arthropods blocking his sight and stinging his cheeks. He tried to see his feet, he stamped them but could only see flies. He saw he was in a desert, the flies had stirred up the sand, or was there a terrible storm as well? If only he could rise above them; he felt a very hot sun. He yelled and started walking towards someone far off. As he got closer layers of his skin were stripping off, he was a little lethargic then he had a bit of a headache then he felt he was burning and then he was bones; all his flesh had been sand blasted, he was a skeleton and suddenly he fell at the feet of a girl, a psychology student he had once dated.

"Depend on me, love me, I will help you, look there are no more flies, promise to follow me, I will make you whole" she said.

He crawled back into the sandstorm of flies, he went to the heart of it and, grabbing hold of them, he swung them all around. Now they were all one, joined. He threw himself and them across the desert plains and wished them good and looking down he stood on his own two feet in a pair of levi's and a white t-shirt. It was sunny, he turned around and there half a mile away was a blue ocean; he fancied a swim.

The rest of the night Pete was stuck in this lucid dream, one he would not remember. This wasn't anything abnormal for him, he often spent long nights travelling over foreign, beauty endowed landscapes or engaging in some strange visual allegories that were meant to mean something to Pete. Most of a great lesson should have been learnt. The locusts were meant to imply changes but Pete beat them away by replying they meant jack shit and explaining the lesson only pointed at a transitional phase he was going through and thanking them anyway. Thus would ensue a conversation about its merits. Pete enjoyed this life, but he was stuck in this place and the deaf saw all his activities as foolishness. There was though one who had no respect for the community as Pete perceived it, he had given Pete the locust dream and he had not been successful in his aim, an aim of evil malice. Pete woke up.

"I'll get you." A voice came out of the wall. He put this voice to the back of his mind among files labelled threats, ones that would remain untouched unless some surreal spirit archaeologist might dig them up decades later, maybe trying to understand Pete. Pete laughed. Turn the other cheek was the phrase. People had rarely ever got to Pete - he had nothing they could take to provoke an action, he did not rely on any guidance that could lead to some debt, he was more a scavenger. He dozed for another hour or so contemplating it. He had nothing better to do, he wasn't going anywhere in this hospital.

Mickey the nurse walked up to the other nurses outside

Pete's door and said something to them out of Pete's earshot. One of them came into the room and opened the curtains. He said,

"Get up. There will be coffee in a bit. It's ten o'clock, I'll maybe have a game of scrabble with you later. Eh?"

It was dull, usual weather for the time of year and country. It never bothered Mickey, the weather. Pete hauled himself out of the bed and into the shower cubicle; a nice hot shower. He sat on the ground and made all the hot water fall on his scalp. After ten minutes of this he got out and shouted out for Wolfie; he couldn't find him. He wanted a shave but the nurses wouldn't let him have razor blades.

"Have one later" he thought. He got changed and walked towards the door,

"I'm ready." The guy in the next room was jabbering to Mickey about how he felt about being "imprisoned" in this place.

"All right man?" said Pete.

Pete watched him, he didn't say hello, he just walked past and the nurses took him to the canteen where he was free to sit where he wanted. He got a cup of tea and a couple of "Nice" biscuits and sat beside his neighbour.

"Hi, my name's Pete, what's yours?"

The guy looked at him and didn't reply.

"His name's Steven." a voice said in Pete's mind.

"Ah, it's Steve, horrible place this huh?"

The voice again said, "You should be careful."

Pete wondered about this muteness; this guy seemed okay. He listened cautiously; the only thing he could hear was the starting of a gale whipping the windows outside.

"I am here, I am going to get you." The gale pattering sounded like a voice. Pete didn't like this, tried not listening to the wind. He looked at the spoon on the table. The metal colour of the spoon gave him a cold feeling, he put it in the cup and tapped the side of it. The sound made him feel sick, his head was swirling,

"How long you been here for?" Pete talked to no one psychically like he did with Wolfie, he did not expect a reply, a kind of telepathy (Pete hated that word, telepathy) then…

"You just got in last night. I have been here two nights, I have been in here before, though when I was here it was in a different building." So the guy could speak.

Pete tried to think bright, he looked over at his new friend, but he only felt he was doing so to get away from this phantom, this panic that seemed to be chasing him. His new friend's eyes were searching him. Pete felt a sliver of terror. Everywhere he looked he thought he was just doing so to dispose of this wretched way. He wanted to disappear and come back later when it had gone.

This had happened to Pete before, being trapped, all he had to do was wait it out, but this emerging spirit was a heavyweight, it was trying to make him let it live in his mind. It was trying to enslave him! The others had just wanted to hurt him.

"Yeah, see that guy?" Pete saw him nod at a nurse with a beard who was contentedly listening to the other nurses chat.

"He's called Bobby, a complete cunt."

"Yeah" Pete slurred. Voices were swarming round him, he didn't like it and he didn't like being around other patients who he reasoned could join in, but was he being paranoid? The voice would stop then, it seemed to force Pete to visualize that other patients were supporting them. But when he tried to see if they were he couldn't tell, they were dishing out actions from their mind but the soul and the body are not linked. They just sat at the tables.

"Bastards" Pete thought. A pickle; again from experience Pete knew not to respond, he would not notice in time. But such a period would return; Pete took that for granted.

He stared at Steve feeling any emotion he had was draining from his soul. He tried to feel some sentiment; he only heard some angry teacher's voice saying he was going to "do him over" and that he "had got mixed up with the wrong people" and that he "didn't know who he was messing with" along with a barrage of other ominous clichés. Pete returned to a stoical resistance but he hadn't given up.

"Pete, the master of his own reality." This seemed fickle at that time.

"Go fuck yourself," he said under his breath. Steve had been watching him and motioned,

"Why are you here, what's up?" Nearly everyone had left having finished dinner. Out of the nurses only his guards remained. Pete replied:

"I get down some times." He looked around; these mothers weren't going to leave. The nurses shouted over, Pete and Steve put the cups and an unfinished biscuit on a cart for the kitchen workers to clean and were followed back to their secured rooms. It was now late morning and everyone at the hospital had been up and were no longer sluggish from sleep aided by medication.

"Okay boys, scrabble" said Mickey, extending his earlier promise. Pete who was still being 'observed' welcomed the change of focus, at least he hoped it would change his focus and Steven was up for it too. Pete dragged a chair from his room to a table in the small vestibule outside it. There was him, Mickey, Steve and a skinny nurse not much older than Pete. The letters were dealt out but instead of a cordial diversion it was turning out to be a nightmare for Pete who shakily put down the word, "g-i-a-n-t." Mickey congratulated him and he took his go putting down "n-a-v-i-g-a-t-e." using Pete's "n". He landed on a double word score as well as getting points for disposing of all his letters. Pete could sense a lot of movement in the corridor though it wasn't visible to his physical eyesight. When he turned around and looked back into his room it seemed quieter, though would it still be if he went back into it? He was playing scrabble.

Pete stood up; the skinny guy started, and carefully asked where it was he was going. They looked at Pete; he felt his blood pounding through his veins, his eyes darting, chasing something that the rest of them just saw as thin air. He looked at the skinny one and attempted to guide his own vision away from the infernal activities going on in the corridor. He heard him say he didn't care and that it was his (Pete's) fault and to get on with the game (though this conversation was of a telepathic nature).

"Where are you going?" he repeated as Pete was still stood up.

"I need a piss." Pete looked around and quickly walked to his room's toilet. He let everything out of his bladder and devoted a sigh of relief to it. At that moment he escaped from all the negativity that had followed him and he found himself being whispered to: it was Wolfie, he sounded very far away but he was able to say,

"Be careful, I don't know what these guys are capable of, just… wait, OK, OK." and with that he was away. Pete allowed himself a moment of fond appreciation for his friend, then he felt himself in contact with another. It spoke in a sycophantic screech saying, "Hey, hm hm you feel that for me too, hm hm, hey everyone, look." and Pete could see and feel a plethora of other fiendish spirits rushing to him. Pete struggled to explain them away - he wasn't offended with any of them, they caused violent gestures, being visual like this it was harder to ignore, it caused him to be dealing with people he did not want any part of. He blanked the lot out of his mind to the best of his ability and exited the room, very unsteady.

"Right, my go?" he stammered. Steve was in good spirits; Mickey was showing a rather benevolent demeanour while also giving the impression that he was enjoying himself, and the skinny one wasn't very good at the game and was stuck with five vowels and didn't hide his puzzlement.

"Yeah, you're up." Pete felt amusement as he watched himself sit down and fix his letters, "m-o-o-k-t-a-c" he had in front of him. "That's not a word" he thought, tittering. He went for "h-o-o-k", and stuck his hand into the bag and got his replacement letters. It was Mickey's go again. Now Pete felt rooted to the spot, his thoughts deduced that the spectres knew where he was; shit. He searched for Wolfie, he searched for dead relatives, friends, there was no one.

He could see them all fooling with Steve, where were the nice ones Pete had met? They were trying to make Steve's soul shadowed to trick him to exchange something or make a silly bet for his soul and it seemed to him that he was in great danger. Pete gaped at him and whispered,

"Don't do it." Mickey was putting down his letters and trying to get Pete to talk. He said, "Are you all right?" He knew the answer was negative, but asked Pete this as a sort of illustration that people should live in a reality and also though he'd asked this many times and failed he slightly hoped that someone would give him an explanation for the insanity that he saw plague so many people in his line of work.

The game ended. Mickey 210, Pete 189, Steven 105 and the skinny guy 88. Pete was back in his room, he could have sat with the nurses but he was kind of fed up having to watch himself, no unnecessary bother. He was also again a little shaken. He watched himself in this shaken state and didn't know what to tell himself. He called out in his mind for help, but someone else was watching him and only people who disliked Pete, who had it in their disposition, partied with this poor unfortunate, keeping him to themselves, molesting him, but Pete had fortitude.

Chapter 6
An Unjust Reward

Nurse Mickey was in the nurses' station, he was hunched over a table where his coffee sat. Across, standing beside the sink, was another nurse, he'd been working this place since Mickey had started and had hardened from all these 'basket cases'. The mind was so temperamental, one faulty dopamine receptor and all sorts of crazy stuff could happen; paranoia; death-like depression; hyper mania; he'd seen it all, insanity. He likened it to life - him a boat on calm waters going straight to his destination, the patients in choppy waters sailing around in circles in the same place. He saw himself getting on in life, them in a kind of paralysis.

"How are you, hard day at the office man?" said Scot to Mickey.

Mickey walked beside him and put his cup in the sink. Replying he said,

"You know it was strange; you know that new patient, the one Doctor Jobes just brought in under observation, he was battling against something, I mean the guy's mad, whispering and that, but it's pure weird, unsettling."

"Yeah I'll check him out tonight, chill man, I'll keep an eye on him, believe me I've seen it all before." And he left Mickey (his shift starting) and Mickey made another coffee.

He was now alone. The coffee was too hot, he tipped a bit into the sink and put more milk in. It turned white.

It tasted of 'fortnight' coffee, it was too weak (two week). He cursed and poured it down the basin and looked to leave. He paced around, it was dark outside and light in here.

"You're weak" he thought he heard, he went towards the door then he sat down, his head in his hands. No one came into the room.

"Why am I here?" he pondered, but when he really thought about it where should he be? He thought about his wife, could she see him? He felt a chill, a kind of panic. She couldn't, she wasn't able to, she was miles away. He could only see a picture of himself, his thoughts were pulsing away from him like heat from the sun. He couldn't focus on anything else, he was bathed in his own fear; it disgusted him. He tried to snap out of it by looking at the window, but it was dark and he only saw his own reflection and the lit room.

He looked at himself, he was smiling. He asked himself "Was that him smiling?" He concluded, "it wasn't."

"It's the end of your shift, go home, enough of this weird shit" he coached himself. He bounded out of the staff tea room; one of younger new patients smiled at him at the vending machine, he temporarily composed himself and said, "Hello young man, I hope you'll be going to the occupational therapy with Sian?" and on down the corridor he went. Usually when he left the ward and his temperament was calm, he would be leaving the place as he imagined it was - a place of therapy, a place where he had good relationships with his colleagues and the patients. And he'd be going home to a kind wife and privacy, privacy where he could relax. All of these good strands of his life were being burnt away. He tried to resurrect them. He was struck dumb. The place had become a savage arena and he cursed it, but where was he going and, even worse, how was he going to get there?

He walked past Scot by the room Pete was in and waved, imagining it was all usual, then telling himself it was and as he pushed the door he dropped everything, any emotions he still had like a bag of groceries, shit, fuck, it was still going on.

Outside he grabbed his keys and knifed the car key into the door and threw open the door. He revved the engine and the radio came on. He sped off. He was on the main road. He'd forgotten to turn on his lights, so he flicked them on, yes he was getting away . He forgot about everything, he was the master of his own ship, getting away.

The ship "Nile" was beside him. Calm and chasing him, beside him, he glanced over at Nile, Nile waved, they smiled, "Go straight ahead." he heard. Nile pointed straight ahead, he put his foot down and sped up, it was a race, faster, he went straight into a brick wall and he lay dead in the wreckage, blood seeping over the dashboard. Shit, he'd been tricked. He could hear the person who had caused his death laughing, saying to a cohort,

"Did you hear Mickey was on the radio - and the steering wheel and the dashboard!" He howled with laughter. Mickey wished he'd thought of his wife before he died, his Linda, he'd never look into her eyes again, he hoped someone would hurt that Nile, he heard the word "yes!" and he was back in the ward, at the front of Pete's bed.

"Get that guy." Pete heard him and said "Okay." Scot watched him. He asked who it was Pete was talking to, Pete didn't answer. It was a long night for Pete, he couldn't think what to do, no ideas, he didn't even dream, he knew who to get, it was that spirit, the one who'd been bothering him during scrabble, it had no faith in life, it empirically demonstrated that fact by butchering those who were content, those who had a taste for the living water of righteousness, the sort of spirituality that couldn't be corrupted. Mickey's problem had been that he wasn't prepared to die for any belief, he told himself nothing was worth dying for. And when he died he asked why he had been killed with such guile? - no particular reason, Mickey began to think this sucked, he envied people who had perished for things like religion but he didn't feel completely empty, he would try and shine, shine.

And there was Pete who watched out of his door which was ajar as Scot was brought to the phone at the nursing station. He came back visibly shaken and beckoned the other two nurses. He said that it had been Linda on the phone, they knew her from parties, Mickey always spoke of her with great pride and love; her the mother of their unborn child. They had been present when Mickey first told them how he'd met this Linda; then he had got engaged and eventually they had seen them as the happy couple married the Christmas just passed.

"Mickey's had an accident." he said in a whisper.

"What, he had what?" This caused him to raise his voice.

"He's had an accident." Pete heard him too this time, it confirmed and explained the apparition. Scot explained what had happened quietly. One of the nurses observed,

"It must have been the brakes." It was now about an hour to the end of their shift, it went terribly slowly for them. Pete fell asleep and had a dream, a dream of feelings where he was dealing with things. The next shift had started and everyone was really cut up, they always got the patients up at 9 o'clock for breakfast and Pete was beginning to stir in anticipation of this call. He often just lay there, but he'd get up after much badgering, he thought. Two things got him up though; first Wolfie came to him saying he must leave, you have a task, and the second was him realising that it wouldn't be Mickey waking him up, as he sat up. Mickey was dead.

A nurse looked over at him and didn't see Pete's usual visage of weary lethargy. He acknowledged him by saying that something awful had taken place and (he waited in the hope that a long pause would help things) then he gave a mumble like he was considering a point and he yelled to Pete's neighbour Steve and told sleepy Steve he had something “heavy” to tell him.

“Listen, Mickey’s dead, bad car crash.” During the morning and over cereal and hot tea the staff and the patients kept separate vigils in a desperately morbid act to commiserate over Mickey. Pete didn’t really bother with the collective mood of his peers. A mood that would confront Mickey with a wall of silence. The purpose of mourning, Pete thought, was to ignore the new spirit to send them on their way. He had a lump in his throat. And Pete had a job to do, he’d got all the kicks out of this damned place that he was going to get, it was time to leave, and he started to seek an incorruptible goal, something that when found would be his motivation to get out of here.

Was it to get Nile? It was more than that, it was to bring Nile back to God, away from his prey, along with anyone else he bumped into on the way, he thought bravely. He gazed around the room at the patients and the nurses, a half full cup of tea in front of him and beside him he looked at Steve who was disturbed and mixed-up. Steve looked at Pete who looked perplexed and bewildered. He said in a groan to Steve that shit was fucked up.

Pete began thinking of where this dickhead Nile was. He began to think where Mickey was, was he okay? Pete knew it was a war field out there past this fabled Hades. But in Pete’s life he had things down to a tee, part of this was that he knew what he would do for eternity, no mean feat. All he had to do was not get too involved in society and love his neighbour and Jesus; best stick to what you know. Pete was reminded of the social commentator from a long time ago who decided that people should give up basic rights for protection. It was reflected in modern day by the fact that people paid taxes to a higher power, who this higher power was was debated fervently among the people, was it a secretive illuminati or was it just the prime minister, they followed some thing or someone. But whoever the king was in this day it was meant to lead to a quiet life. Pete was thinking about this in an awkward, strained way.

But back to Mickey and the demon Nile - to them when they began their death it was quickly discovered that this so called leviathan (the thing Pete had been thinking of) of the world they came from was out of the window. Many of the dead spent a lifetime trying to get or establish one back, some legal protection that never materialized. People who didn’t bother with this false pursuit didn’t necessarily have a bad life but they risked many things, most of which were dangerous to the extreme, but then you only die once. Like some people in a sort of desperation wanting to "follow" them! Or people wanting to enslave them, people like Nile (his numbers growing daily). When there were people offering to follow you being responsible for a person it quickly drained one's energy; the power, they sucked and prised one's compassion. Most people setting out had experienced both at some time, after all you had to learn.

"No, it does not mean death" Pete thought, getting up from the table. This knowledge was a sort considered subversive and was deplored by the silent majority of the living world, but often in a practical way because it usually meant "contact" with things that the doctors and many people classed conveniently as madness, insanity. But Pete was soon to meet another who was above this bullshit Pete had emerged from and that was the Voodoo man. At the minute though his only associate was Wolfie, a ghost that had adjusted well to life.

"Hello young man."

Pete turned around. It was Melanie, a staff nurse under the doctors. She said to him in a matter of fact way that he was being relegated to semi confinement. This meant, she indicated with her hand in a sweeping motion, that he was free to go where he liked in the ward on his own. What was in the ward? Well, Pete got up, he looked at Steve (Steve had been missed by Melanie) and said,

"Did you hear that? Hey man, no bother, I will call round, we're still part of the same bullshit." Pete stood up, he threw a spiritual "YEE HA!" towards Wolfie, who went towards it and he watched Pete walk out of the cafeteria leaving Steve. Halfway down the corridor Pete and Wolfie acknowledged two inmates by saying,

"...in the same boat." Then Pete looked for another "same boat" and walked round the corner to the smoking room. Pete didn't smoke. The room was clouded with smoke and four people looked up, not talking but enjoying their smoke. There was a hi-fi playing the rap of "Ice-T." Pete listened to the beats and turned, exploring the rest of this place. He walked past many rooms. This hospital was modern, in the fact that the patients all had their own rooms (some wards had big dorms). He walked down past rooms on each side. Their doors were shut, but they had windows so the nurses could carry out suicide watches while everyone was asleep. Pete got to the bottom; there was a pay phone and a television room. He went in.

It was a small room with armchairs. MTV was on. Pete took a seat and looked at the others sitting there. He said "Right" to the guy across the room and got chatting. The guy across the room was a university graduate, intellectual, he was amicable and explained that he was manic depressive and Pete deduced that he didn't really mind being here, having everything with him that he needed, he could be at home, it really didn't matter. He left him to figure things out and turned to the other guy. A nurse popped his head into the room and ticked everyone off on a clipboard.

"So hey man, where you from?" said Pete. The guy looked up. He looked like a bit of a chav, but he was quite obtuse.

"I'm from the outer estate." he spoke, naming a rough area of City 29 (the city Pete lived in) and said his name was Keith.

"Yeah man, I dig that." Pete named a drug dealer who, it turned out, they both knew. Then he continued,

"Shame about Mickey, huh?" Keith motioned his hands in a circular way and Pete thought about it more instead of giving a vocal reply. Wolfie flew in. Pete wondered about Nile, he wasn't about so he said, carrying on their interaction,

"How come you're here?" he waited to hear some convoluted psyche jargon people said to explain things regarding mental illness. For Pete nothing really had an explanation, in fact after long periods of visions and devilish conversations he just said "fuck it." He drifted into a powerful day dream;

"I want to be pulled out of this proverbial hat that is my life, one controlled by the master, the ego. One life which replied to anything should only be thanked by a physical act otherwise it is dismissed as a product of one's own intelligence. Here is the life of the ego with its plethora of egotistical illnesses!" Anyhow, Pete waited then wondered what the hell he had just been talking about…

"You know how it is mate, too much toking, too much acid when it was around, but fuck it, I never really much fancied work, most of my friends like, it's sound you know…" and Keith's words petered out in a mixed up string of nostalgia. Pete relaxed. He turned to look towards the door; there was a hippy looking guy standing there waiting for acknowledgement.

"Keith ma man, I've come to visit you." His name was Voodoo man. The university guy whom Pete met upon entering had grown agitated during the ensuing conversation and got up and left. This Voodoo man talked with a strange kind of slur and Pete looked into the void at Wolfie tittering in his mind. Voodoo man paused and he actually looked up at Wolfie. Pete saw this. Neither knew what to do. Pete just thought "fuck it" and slouched into the seat listening to the talk from the guys' neighbourhood slightly amused. The three chewed the fat.

The talk centred around strange trips that had been happening like someone smoking a quarter of ganja a day, while both of them said it screwed them up, neither longer took drugs. About their mate "Wiener" getting pissed at the local club and getting the shit knocked out of him by the local heavy who had in turn once had his drink spiked with a trippy ecstasy and ended up stripped in the car park where he proceeded to shit himself, this they told for Pete's benefit as it had happened last year and was not new to them. Keith also asked the visitor if any of his friends knew of his whereabouts, as apart from Voodoo man knowing of his admittance to this place, it was secret. The reply was negative. Keith got up and said,

"Smoke." They walked out the door, past the payphone, then by an avenue of closed doors (more bedrooms, of which there where many in Meadow bank) past the nurses at reception and there was the smoking room at the other end beside which was Pete's room and also Steve's room.

"Whatcha Steve." Steve was looking at the comings and goings and was sat up on top of his bed and said in an excited mutter that things were a-okay. Pete and his new friends entered the smoking room. There were three other guys there and the television was showing a channel five quiz (not like any of them were watching it though).

Keith said, "Right?" with an underlying tone that said he was interested in the others. One of the three smokers looked up and said "hi" with a nervous stutter. The other two just stared at the wooden floor. Pete slumped into a high backed seat and grinned, breathing in his mind much happiness, then he returned to the room though most of the happiness stayed with him. Pete and Voodoo man begin rolling their bacci, both using the same American brand, while Keith lit up a king size cig and there was a moment of quietness which Pete being the outsider felt slightly uncomfortable in sharing, so he asked Voodoo man what he did.

It was noticed by Voodoo man that Pete felt "uncomfortable" and this took over his silence. Someone pounced, Voodoo man gazed at Pete leaving others in his mind behind and threw in an infernal ghost who had frequented him and his own mind the odd time. Now he had something to share, exhaling a plume of smoke and coughing at the irony of his intellect; Voodoo man smiled, though Pete who perceived this spirit was not lost to it nor did he let himself be fickle to this hippy invoker beside him. The ghost returned with a bump. Pete watched with a dull fascination as the hippy Voodoo man didn't know quite what to do… shit happens.

Pete looked round the smoke room. Keith had been oblivious to the suspect exchange and the other smokers were zonked out on powerful medication so did not notice anyhow. The ward was getting on with the business of the fucked up; the depressives; the delusional; the schizophrenics; their invisible entourages and the nurses who stopped things going loco.

"So hey man, bet you're glad you're not in this fucking shithole." Pete motioned.

"Well I've been up you know, visiting my nigger Keith here." And so that was the first introduction Pete had to the Voodoo man.

Later. He gripped Pete's hand and shook it up and down while murmuring a respect he extended to every person he met. Oh to be known.

While he said goodbye to Pete and Keith the head nurse, Scot and the consultant were also discussing something that would shape Pete's destiny.

"What do you think, I mean now he's on medication?" said the doctor. (He just wanted an opinion.) Being a doctor he knew the clinical progression of these people's behaviour once on, and for that case off, medication. He had seen hundreds of Pete's.

"I think his being here a little longer, say a month, should do the trick. Get him back into the grind of things…"

"You mean the positive symptoms, his damaged intellect, underlying manias. On the other side his negative ones like lack of sleep or depression seem to be below average in manifestation. Okay Scot watch him, watch him and tell me if there's any change, principally if he becomes withdrawn or if you notice any other displays or exhibitions of the positive symptom side of things." That was the end of them talking about Pete, they moved on to another patient.

The next month was spent listening to the radio, playing pool and card games and, every day, drinking numerous hot beverages with scones. Keith had left about ten days before Pete got to leave, he went home to his parents who lived on an estate outside the city limits, but where would Pete go? He'd never see Keith again. Pete was going to one of the trust's hostels. He would "take part in the cooking and cleaning rotas and go to the mental health day centre close by at least 3 times a week." It could have been worse, once he got the aforementioned activities over he was free to do as he wished as long as he returned sober and back at the curfew, which was reasonable. With no work to do and new people to meet he would have a fine time.

Meanwhile at the Stevens ward people came and went and the nurses carried on playing scrabble and watching and occasionally restraining the disturbed and other patients.

Chapter 7

Pete never looked back on that awful hospital nor did he run into any of the nurses or the inmates.
All is normal on the outside....

A social worker ushered Pete in, into a 2 story hostel in the leafy outer suburbs of the south, where he was cordially greeted by the hostel manager.

"Hi Pete, I'm Padraic. Ah you've got your stuff, good." Though he directed this to the social worker more. The social worker stood back and Padraic allowed himself to be followed up a nicely carpeted, banistered staircase that reached the first floor.

"Ah here we are." He had a key and opened the door (number 3) and gave the key to Pete. They went inside. There was a bed beside a radiator and window, a cabinet and a wardrobe. The walls were painted a pastel green colour.

"Now this is great." said the social worker, "I'll leave you to it and if you need me don't hesitate to phone, Padraic has my number and most of the forms are filled in." They both looked at each other then as he left he said,

"I'll have that coffee some other day, see you Paddy." and he left. Pete looked around and Padriac motioned him into the corridor. He said he'd show him around.

They walked down the hall and stopped outside a door and he gave it a rap. An extremely thin lady in her twenties opened it and before she could speak, who knows maybe she wouldn't have spoken, Padraic introduced her to Pete. Her name was Rhona. She gazed into the air and muttered something inaudible and Padraic said in a cheery tone that he'd see her in half an hour and that it was her "turn to cook tonight."

He showed Pete the communal shower room of which there were two (though only one had a bath) on this floor. Beside the top of the stairs there was a smoking room. It wasn't yet night but the ash trays were nearly overflowing. There were a couple of individuals in it watching "Joanna" - one of those daytime television programmes where all the guests are incredibly stupid. Pete strode in front of Padriac and poked his head round the door.

"Hey how's it going, my name's Pete." Pete looked at each of them with eye contact, kind of watching them but only so he could react in an amicable way which usually worked when meeting new people.

"Yeah my name's Ryan, mm hello… ah." The other guy stood up and bounded forward and gripped his hand saying with a smile of enjoyment,

"Mine's Bob, Joe Bob." Pete liked this Joe Bob and Ryan too; he was about to sit down with them when his shoulder was tapped and Padriac said he needed to show him a few more things.

"You can see each other at dinner." They walked down to the bottom floor and into the kitchen and over to the fridge. There was a sheet of paper inside a clear folder. It was some kind of rota with people's names on it with columns and ticked boxes.

"This my friend is the rota of chores, everybody mucks in, we all take turns at cooking and cleaning…" and he continued to talk. Pete had no questions.

Pete passed Rhona on the stairs and she brushed passed him at a quick pace then slowed down for the last couple of steps. Pete wasn't insulted. He hauled his bag up and threw it up onto the air, it landed on his bed. This bed had been slept on by many others and Pete felt pleased it was now his. He looked out of the window and saw a leafy branch of a tree and he turned round, closing the door.

Pete took the opportunity to throw a "hi" to Wolfie the dead one. Wolfie showed he was glad to see him and then retreated to a part of Pete's mind that Pete wasn't thinking of then disappeared contented and a little thrilled that he emerged into such a nice place which was also a reason Pete had summoned him.

Now the chance to meet Ryan and Joe Bob re-presented itself again, he walked in to the smoking room and sat down. They were listening to a golden oldie radio station coming through the freeview on television. Pete observed this and started to roll some bacci in a small size cigarette paper. He pondered about the times he would have been burning some low grade blo into it. He turned away from the nostalgia but one of the others spoke.

"Yeah I used to smoke that shit, wipe out" mused Joe Bob. Had Joe Bob heard what Pete was thinking?

"That's just hand rolling tobacco" said Ryan. Ryan had not heard.

"I know man" retorted Joe bob. Pete looked up and smiled then offered them some tobacco. But the answer was no. Ryan sat looking into nothing and Joe Bob produced a cigarette and positioned it in front of Pete to say thanks but no thanks.

Pete said to himself, "If this is hostel life, I dig it." Joe Bob raised his cigarette and said, "Touche." The rest of that time was mostly a blur. Joe Bob told him about a life that had been rather uneventful, he had been born into a family that although not very poor had not been rich either. He had received average grades in school, but as his life had reached a turning point in his last year at comprehensive… (he continued).

"I felt like education was not only guiding my intellect, also my beliefs; I was being led into a world of intolerance, intolerant of people who don't give a fuck, yeah, (he kind of snarled) I mean being part of social reality makes you deaf, so I went onto the weed and then the voices began, ya know what I mean…" His story was much the same as Pete's except Joe Bob's voices gave him a lot of room and admired him, Pete's often did not. They both thought this was strange. Pete liked him. Ryan was now struggling to look at nothing and said, "I'm going for dinner." They followed him down. It was potato waffles and frozen quiche (Rhona's special). Three other people dined with Pete that day. There was Danny, a withdrawn guy in his fifties, who when he made eye contact gave off an air of contempt and quickly retreated into his thoughts. Then there was Abigail, a woman with dirty blonde plaited hair. She did not look at Pete when he came in and she mumbled with a slight grin when Joe Bob said "hi."

"Hey Abigail, after tea we're going to show Pete here the local, eh Pete?" Another guy called Dwight asked eagerly, "Can I come?"

"Sure." said Joe Bob. Padraic had been standing leaning against the door frame; now he walked towards the table.

"It's your turn to wash, Dwight" he said helpfully. Dwight looked younger than his age and had a big grin on his face.

"Don't worry, we'll wait." said Ryan.

Chapter 8
Out to the Local

Ryan, Pete, Joe Bob, Abigail and Dwight slipped out into the night. Most people were still eating their tea and there was not much traffic, and they strolled past lamp posts and bus stops not seeing any passers by. A scuffed blue sierra with a strange aerial sped by at 25 mph in third gear. Inside the car it was smoky from a recently stubbed out cigarette, and there was another guy apart from the driver. Their suits had been bought a long time ago, no longer sharp; the original colour of the driver's suit had faded to a greyish black and to a greyish blue in the case of the passenger.

The walkers were not aware of the conversation in the strange car. "This is 259 calling. Delta 4 and squad are sauntering down the road, there's the new member if you want to listen in, they will be at the Golden Horse bar in five."

"Yeah we know who that is, his name's ...." and the babble continued. But to the rest of the world on a first look they were just a group of five friends going for a drink.

And there was yet another person with a more than casual interest in a certain member of the group. He was our old friend Voodoo man. He had his arm slung round the back of a three seater as he watched the five enter the pub. His eyes met Pete's as Pete made his way to the bar. Pete paused as the others went to get their drinks. Pete spoke first.

"Oh hi."

"Yeah hi Pete." Pete perceived this welcome.

"Just out with new friends." Pete looked at Voodoo man and smiled, and then at Joe Bob and the rest of them (who he was looking forward to getting to know).

"Come on over and sit with me and my friends."

Voodoo man's demeanour did not alter, he just sat and gazed at Pete. Pete glanced back into his eyes. Voodoo man raised himself and said,

"OK."

The friendly barman (who knew Pete's friends) pulled 5 pints of special and a whisky and soda for Abigail; then took a collection of pound and fifty pence coins and dinged the till. All the drinks were set down on one table. The beer mats were already soggy and torn.

"Everyone, this is..." and Pete gave Voodoo man's name. Ignoring the room Voodoo man looked at each member of the group with equal interest, and smiled, suggesting he wanted them to think he was pleased to see them.

"So anyway," Dwight continued, "I saw the new 'After Dark' slasher movie; it was mental." He was getting excited, he appeared oblivious to the vibes from the Voodoo man, "They must have killed, I dunno, a hundred people in the first quarter." He spat while he talked and Pete, Joe Bob, Ryan and Abigail all nodded with an irrelevant delight. Having finished, Dwight sipped the froth off his beer.

Voodoo man thought, "Fucking prick", and Pete and Joe Bob gave a look of pain in his direction. Dwight felt he'd forgotten what he was going to say. Next Abigail, who was unaware, began humming happily. The barman put on some sixties pop music, it made everyone smile. Ryan started to sing.

"So the people round this district are okay?" Pete asked.

"I'm not from here, I am from outside town, near Whitdale. Usually there's no bother, but this bar gets a bit loud on the Sunday folk music get together. You can hear it from the hostel." It was Ryan that said this.

"Don't have much contact with anyone outside the hostel" someone chipped in. Most of the tenants had once had testing mental health conditions. They had spent "time" in various institutions. They were in high spirits and had been discharged recently like Pete. Pete too was in high spirits and could see the joy in them. From far off Wolfie smiled too.

Pete was taking a break and had quit thinking about his future for now. These cats he had met today were okay and that was all he needed. He just wanted to chill and gather himself. He was not going back to the Stevens ward, ever.

Then he heard a growl of horror, no one else heard. He had left the Voodoo man to himself. But now during his ponderings a part of Pete's nature had been attacked - his psyche had been slapped would be a better description.

Pete was suspicious. The others sat, they were giggling at a silly joke that Voodoo man was recounting. Pete tried to meet Voodoo man's gaze (but the nerve of this guy). This gaze was returned by a look that said he thought Pete had been listening to his story. Pete, frustrated, saw through him. He continued to pull at Pete's consciousness as he talked. Pete glared at him but the others laughed along with the joke. Pete had let his mind be ripped, in the future he'd be wary about this guy's company. But maybe this would not be enough. Voodoo man's soul seemed to be inside Pete. Pete did not want the others to know what was happening. He nodded at Joe Bob, who immediately strangely keyed in with what was happening. A shutter came down. All was gone.

Voodoo man had stopped talking. Abigail was trying to blow bubbles through a straw in her whisky and soda. Ryan and Dwight were laughing. Pete no longer felt invaded. But his brain had had a rush of blood, his head had been left with a stupefying fuzzy feeling.

He called out to Wolfie who said, “I am coming!” and he rushed to Pete's aid. Pete felt normal. Wolfie disappeared. Where did Wolfie go? Joe Bob did not know where either, he had been watching this small battle from the start.

The other possible culprit, Voodoo man, sat with a gleaming expression on his face making it look like he was enjoying the taste of his special beer. Wolfie was gone.

For the rest of the night Pete sipped at his beer slowly and in the two hours they had all been there, he had only had two pints. Another slow drinker that night was the Voodoo man who had quit trying it on with Pete. He had not heard it in speech or in the mind but Joe Bob had made it clearly certain that Voodoo man was to “leave.” Voodoo man rushed away quietening his mind, for now.

“Just a retard with some eccentric extraordinary fluke skills, leave him alone. Fucking mental patients” thought Voodoo man.

“Well it was nice meeting you although I forget your name” Abigail giggled to Pete's friend. A fare helping of ‘dutch’ courage backed her up, it was quite out of character, that was a lot for her, she was normally so painfully shy.

“Cool, I'll call if I am ever round this way again” he replied. Pete knew this was a lie but he would keep the option open if he ever had use of this person, although he could not think why. The others had already walked off. Dwight and Ryan had already forgotten the Voodoo man.

They rang the hostel's electric doorbell. Padraic opened the door, he was talking to a bouncy woman with ginger hair. He told her,

“And this is our new tenant Pete. And Pete this is our night worker Louise. Now it's the end of my shift and, hey you guys, it's quite late, so don't be making this a habit. I know you're only having fun but studies show this could be bad for your recovery." The residents thought this was meaningless. Padriac continued,

"We will talk about some other stuff tomorrow, Pete, my man." Then he left.

Pete had cheered up. Not yet had he heard, or felt, something was wrong with Wolfie.

"I fancy a kebab but I'd settle for a bowl of cornflakes" Pete said to Louise.

"I'm sorry but the kitchen's closed. It's too late, we've found kitchen noise keeps the other residents awake." Then she smiled. The others had gone upstairs to the smoking room.

"So you work the nights?"

"Yes, I've worked here for three and a half years. I am employed in case any resident has a problem during the night. It is not the most sociable of hours but I have read at least a hundred romantic novels! I've also seen the late night telly such as the costume jewellery channel." She smiled as if she felt this was time well spent.

"So no chance of anything to eat then?" Pete enquired.

"Well seeing as you're new…"

Chapter 9
You Sit in the Car Outside

The blue sierra had only one passenger; a man was talking to his wife on a mobile phone. His colleague was down the road at a chip shop in a queue for fish and chips and a couple of lemonades. It was late and the place would be closed in half an hour. The woman eventually called out his number,

"Number two-one-two," which was pointless as there was nobody else in the shop.

"That's me." said Connor. The petite teenager at the till poured on a load of salt and vinegar. "And anything else?"

"Ketchup, thank you." She handed over the two fish suppers plus drinks. The bag had 'tasty fish and chips' written on it. The man now sauntered back to the car. He disliked eating take-outs in the car. They left a rank smell all next day. They also made his fingers greasy, and he knew they helped put on the weight he was trying to lose. He opened the door and reflected happily for a second that he wasn't in the driving seat cramped behind the steering wheel.

The radio was on, 105fm, the night bird hour. His wife often put a request in for him, he liked "Dire Straits."

"Here's yours Bazza." said Conner. They did not talk while they ate. It was a responsible job they were in. They had been hired from the police force but also it had not been a coincidence that they were in the Masonic order. This had prepared them for life in 'interior defence'. They did not know who gave their orders, nor how their bosses identified these subversives. They were not privy to such information, nor did they really do anything that revealed their overseers' motives. The idea behind their recent days' stake out was to make Pete think he was being followed. That was what the powers that be had told them to do. They were in no doubt that psychically Pete would detect them. Then he would think he was wrong, after all, why else would someone go to all that trouble? But Pete did not give a fuck either way. They'd tried to mess with him before on Stevens ward. Pete's thoughts often rested on important people, powerful people who did not like this invasion; harmless as it was. They'd tracked him and his 'adventures' down (it took a long time) and now they'd nearly got him. They tried to hurt him to shut him up psychically, but he just kept going. Now physical means were being employed to compliment the psychic attacks and that was where Connor and Bazza came in.

Inside the hostel Pete had changed into slippers. He sat in the smoking room with a bowl of cornflakes. The only other resident still up was Danny, he was listening to a sports station that had all the football critics and news of the test cricket match going on in England.

"You into the cricket?" asked Danny.

"No." said Pete. Pete looked at Danny. Danny frowned. Pete had met people like Danny before, they got involved in everything the state carers provided for stimulus of the intellect, the bread and circus idea in today's society. It did not bother him, Pete knew he loved the cinema even though it was subject to their same kind of guidance.

Pete munched his way through the cornflakes. Danny remained lost in thought,

"So Liverpool could play Arsenal but what about the new manager, hmmm I'll listen to the comments on 'Match of the Day' tomorrow, it being a Saturday."

"Do you a wanna roll up?" Pete asked.

"What do you mean?" Pete held a rollie in front of him.

"No thanks, and I hope that lot are out tomorrow so I watch this in peace."

Pete mused about what had brought Danny into this mental health system. Pete had been on weed that he had got off his older brother's mates. He had been happy. He had once lived a nice life, he had gone to a top school and had wanted to do psychology. This aspiration would have taken Pete straight to the hidden side, a working knowledge of the secretive world Pete was now battling, in a controlled way. But when he began to smoke he just thought "Fuck it all! I wanna get high." When he was stoned he pondered the world's social mysteries/conspiracies. In time they began to answer back!

He messed up his end of school exams and ended up doing sociology, 'psychology's poorer cousin.' The mysteries however took away anything that had once been certain in his mind. They became voices and at the time he didn't know who they were. The authorities tried to give him a second chance. To use a cliché, they had wanted to bring him back into the fold, with other students. Pete had not cared for this, he smoked harder and his voices, Pete thought, employed his friends, and maybe they did. They saw what was happening but wanted to be part of the official high flying psychic community.

The men waiting outside the hostel dialled the switchboard in the local military installation. They reported the boy's lights had been turned off. Now they were free to drive off. Pete never seemed to do anything that made their job difficult. All they had to do was sit outside his abode. Originally they felt they had succeeded in making Pete paranoid. Once upon a time he would walk down a street and jump into a hedge, waiting for them to pass. Their superiors would be pleased, so when Pete had checked into a hospital that should have been the end of it. The medication and the stern hand of the nurses and consultants ought to have beaten the problem, but it did not go that way. Pete took to lying in his room messing about with Wolfie and fucking with people. Sometimes Pete even talked to the North Koreans, they were out there in the psychic sphere trying to recruit possible insurgents in other countries, especially western ones. Pete found their attention strangely surreal, a fun game.

Chapter 10
Meet the Handlers

Eight people sat in a conference room on the top floor of a grey building with a rust free metal roof. There was a half moon in the sky and the barracks were deserted apart from some soldiers asleep in their houses, and a guy cleaning up in the nafi.

"Okay, let's start, we've a load of stuff on district 9 and we have a new problem in district 4." The man of African appearance shuffled his papers, all of which read "Secret" and he continued, "Yes district 4, Alaska Drive, only young but could be a problem, yes I'll leave that one for you Curtis."

"Yes, Heather Waring, 10 Alaska Drive. I know the parents, never engaged when young, her helper friends spoke on her level, but she would not engage, then after a year of being a loner she seems to have broken away, no drugs were involved… Yes she's been causing the area quite a lot of trouble, turn her over to the dream team."

The chairperson went through the details of a couple of people who had made regular appearances at these meetings, they included Pete, then there were a couple of 'endgames'.

"Yes good work Carson, Joshua from east district 10 is now under the thumb from one of our "friends." The girl has asserted control over him and he looks up to her in everything he does. And the fourteen year old, Sadie, has told our people in her own way she is going to wait and develop, and be with us. A good prospect."

The meeting came to a conclusion and Nicola, one of the top key "advisors" in a black suit, was the first to push down on the plunger of a cafeteria of Costa Rican coffee and everyone relaxed. The business had been completed. Most of the eight advisors had families to go home to, and it was now late, but the power they had over the destiny of many was addictive.

They chatted, showing off their 'super developed minds' in a way they thought as all knowing, yet beautiful. They hoped their children would never be part of their agenda here. They probably would not, most of them had developed in a most promising way since they were babies. How proud they were as parents.

Pete struggled in bed, it was his first night in a new room but that didn't bother him. He looked down upon the scene that he saw as he turned in the bed. Wofie was far away, he was a galaxy away. Distorting Pete's day had been the awful Voodoo man. He thought about him and there in this scene he saw the demon Nile. The demon was swarming around Voodoo man dissolving his flesh and Voodoo man did not seem to notice. Pete was okay and he wondered if he'd bump into Nile and his new friend. Part of living in this world was you had to be up for anything (for fear only censors the mind). It was this maxim that had brought the key advisors after him. He smiled in his sleep.

Although his sleep was invaded it was still deep. Between 3am and 5:30am a lone person at a military instillation pondered and watched Pete. He slept.

"You'll never amount to anything."

Pete was placed in a nightmare. The ones who loved him all said disapprovingly that this is not the way we love you. Joe Bob was there though Joe Bob's sleep was elsewhere, undetected. All his friends were with him taunting him to become a new sexual being, to use up his energy in a land of perversions, what most people did. It had worked on others.

"We'll help you."

This guy tonight is good Pete thought.

"Back to the dream."

Back to the dream. He allowed himself to be guided, it did not matter that they had him sat at home in a women's dress pleased with it, talking to people. 2 hours later he awoke. The end of a shift, Pete drifted into a different plain; he was emerging to daytime. A man drank a tepid cup of tea.

"Maybe this time I've done it (to himself). You'll be happy (to Pete) a long night of painstaking work." He smiled at his ward, a whole night. Pete got up, rubbed his eyes, smiled at the people looking and said,

"But this is the way I am, go fuck your dress, ha ha ha. Fucking chump." He shifted himself from everyone's view and looked round at his new day, alone again. Happy bordering on ecstatic!

Chapter 11
Where's my Friend?

Four knocks on the door.

"Hi hi Joey Bob, Joe Bobert. Ha ha ha." mocked Padraic. He'd just started his shift and he'd had his brew and now to get the tenants' day started, they needed a firm hand he thought.

"…best not left, never alone."

Joe Bob exclaimed to Padraic -

"Today shall be a good day, I will do two things I don't want to do but it shall be good!" Padraic left and knocked the rest of the other tenants.

"Come on sleepy people." Pete was out the door, following the others a minute ahead already down at the breakfast table. He smiled in his mind, and that gave him a huge Cheshire cat grin, things are the usual screwed up, ha, ha. It was sunny in the street, the leaves were a summer green.

Very suddenly he couldn't quite connect the happiness he felt; it was Wolfie.

"For God's sake help me Pete, I'm not where I was, terror, I dunno where I am!" Wolfie was immediately gone. Pete stumbled to the window sill, a cloud had just crossed the sun and it passed. A clear beam. Pete got to the table but still had time to slag Padraic.

"No danishes Paddo?"

"There's a bakery round the corner."

Pete chumped down a slice of toast with some breakfast juice and thought deeply. Of course he would help his friend, the laws of karma desired it, it went without saying even though they had not known each other long. He'd need to be alone to do this. He got up to go, it was sunny, he'd find a park or somewhere.

"If I could see you for a mo Pete-o?" motioned Padraic. Pete turned and went into the workers' office.

"Well Pete, hello I am just here to welcome you and have a wee chat about what we, well you hope to achieve during your stay." Pete did not have time for this shit but you couldn't let psychic things dominate your behaviour, at least not in front of people like Padraic, the only other person who he didn't mind showing was Joe Bob, a strange guy but totally there.

"So Pete, any hobbies, what do you like?" he said in a slow way keeping eye contact. Pete felt manipulated but from experience he just gave what they wanted, he mused - they never asked for the righteous things, it was always mixed up with negative emotions, that's what the whole telepathy thing is, thoughts towards someone that have no selfish root. The whole of Pete's watchers never understood this, they tried to understand it as a thing alien from one's motivations, tangible. Nor, said Pete, did they care for Jesus. He looked Padraic in the eye and said,

"Well I like reading and the guitar. I like walking by the sea and in forests, I like eating fine food and the cinema, I am also born again and I sometimes meditate, keeps me calm you know?"

"Okay that's interesting, I play a mean guitar myself, what's your axe?" They talked and behind the worker Padraic was quite a nice guy. He told Pete some of the residents went to day centres with craft and wood work, plus a free hot lunch,

"Eh, what about that?"

"I think I'll settle in for a bit and relax after being in Steven's ward for a bit." Pete said tactfully.

"Just so you know the consultants encourage it."

"Thank you." said Pete. He got up and was leaving the room when he was called back in.

"Your turn to cook tonight, if you need any help…"

Pete strode away on his own. Explore, yes that's what I'll do, I'll head south towards the inner suburbs and get a handle on the Wolfie situation. He sent out a positive thought and thought of Wolfie; nothing. He sent out a thought of distress and looked for Wolfie, still nada. What was he playing at, this shit wasn't working, he walked a mile or so. It was sunny and about twenty degrees Celsius, a housewife cleaned her windows. Pete looked back at the previous night, to the exact moment Wolfie went off his radar. Pete took a risk, Wolfie had said,

"I am coming." He imagined he was Wolfie and saw himself and Wolfie at the same time with the same soul saying,

"I am coming." He felt himself falling but dragged at the same time at the same rate as they fell hundreds of feet. He did not land on anything but his dizziness and vertigo became the air around him. A floaty feeling. Then he landed, flat. There was a peculiar feeling, this new land had no horizon, it went on for ever, again. The land was a strange tropical prairie, his legs gave off a weird haze as he ambled, but no Wolfie. Shit. The place was deserted. When he looked up the world flipped him over and he was again looking straight ahead.

All at once a comet flared towards him at waist height. It looked like it had travelled thousands of miles in a fraction of time. It stopped right in front of him. It was a stocky looking man with dark skin and a Buddha's belly.

"Greetings adventurer, you don't belong here, this is a realm, the one you look for is travelling." His eyes acknowledged Pete's impatience but he smiled. Fair enough.

"Right. Good bye." He was back in his body, it was sunny and he assumed it had been this way all the while he was away. He'd been leaning on a tree, he continued his stroll slightly more content than he'd been since leaving the hostel. There was a spiritualist church, the bakery Padraic had mentioned, but mostly apart from last night's bar there were just large detached houses that had been built before the 2nd World War. Pete thought they had aged beautifully with their nice privet hedges and gravel driveways. Now for some lunch, Pete decided.

Chapter 12
Settling in

The others had got back from a day centre. Dwight had made a kite out of wooden dowels and plastic sheets. He had a big grin on his face. Rhona had gone straight to her room. Ryan, Padraic and Danny were in the kitchen. Pete could see them through a hatch that connected the dining room with the kitchen. In the kitchen some bacon was on the go. Tomato soup, that's what I want, Pete thought. Jumping into the kitchen he opened a cupboard. Just a load of cups and coffee.

"Soup, Padraic?"

"Above the cooker." There was only cream of chicken and lentil. Pete liked lentil. He put two tins in a saucepan and soon it was bubbling away.

"Where's Joe Bob?" Abigail asked as she sat at the table.

"He's talking to Olivia." replied Padraic.

"She's one of the day workers, Pete" Abigail blurted. There was enough soup for everyone and Pete dished it out. Joe Bob entered and sniffed the air,

"I hate lentil soup, (sniffing again) But I like bacon, hmm." Padraic took a bowl and sat down at the table too.

"What was Olivia saying? You were in a quiet… anything up?" Ryan said to Joe Bob.

"That bloody day centre, it's not for me, craft and woodwork aren't my hobbies to put it mildly, and they make out it's important therapy that I apparently need, I told her I'm not goin' again." Ryan, Danny, Dwight and Abigail quite liked the day centre, Danny had friends who he played bowls with, Dwight enjoyed doing things with his hands, Abigail liked knitting and talking to old ladies while Ryan liked to chew the fat with the volunteers who helped at the woodwork. But Joe Bob did not like this sort of therapy, he saw it as an intrusion that was meant to modify his behaviour; a place where he was watched. He did not want to be watched by "helpful mental health professionals." Nor did they like him watching them which he'd tried once to alleviate the boredom, they'd walked off and returned with the manager who asked him if he was 'okay.' No now was the right time, change was in the air, he'd been watching people for a long time, that was a talent of his. He could often tell what they thought and unless they were some sort of deviant he liked them. Although they rarely returned his admiration, not even with a simple hello. But this Pete was different!

It was later. Pete was to get a taxi to the local Tesco to buy the ingredients for the week's dinners and a few other things like bread and coffee. All were on a list that Olivia had. She also gave him money and told him to make sure that he got receipts. He waved goodbye to her and opened the front door. It was still sunny. It was nice out in the sun. He waited for a taxi to come. There was a tap on his shoulder, it was Joe Bob. He was going to go with Pete. Pete welcomed the help and company. They began to talk.

"So man, how did you end up in the system?" Pete was going to say but was interrupted as a taxi pulled up and the man wound down his window and beckoned them. Pete got in the front. The Tesco's was about two and a half miles away and like taxi drivers do to save petrol he kept it in fifth gear most of the way with 105fm seeping out through the open window. He had sunglasses on and had the slight smell of body odour.

"£3.50 my friend." Pete paid it and got a receipt like Olivia said. They got a large trolley and pushed it around, picking things up that were on the list. It was all crammed into plastic bags and again they waited for a taxi. They'd didn't have enough time to conclude or start their previous conversation so they talked about music they liked, like 'The Doors.' They also had a common like for techno and trance (electronic music) and they decided that next Saturday they'd go to a top club where 'Dj Nutts' was playing.

"Yeah, cool" they both said in unison. Pete had to get the stuff for dinner sorted so they quit until later. Pete got to work in the kitchen. He didn't eat any old shit, or at least he didn't cook any old shit. Abigail came into the kitchen and sat on the work surface.

"What 'cha cooking Pete?"

"Comfort food Abby, egg fried rice and chicken curry." For the rice he boiled it by putting two centimetres of water in the pan, then when it had shrunk to the same level as the rice he moved it to a low heat and put a plate on top. That would take fifteen minutes. Meanwhile he fried the chicken and set that aside. The rice was nice and sticky, he heated a wok and fried some ginger and garlic for half a minute then he threw in all the rice and stirred. Next a load of soya sauce and Chinese oyster sauce, stirred, and finally eggs. In went the chicken and then the curry sauce. Hey presto. It smelt great.

Abigail helped him put it on plates beside the hatch. Everyone tore into the dinner. Olivia came in;

"That smells great, you'll have to show me how to cook, I am quite awful." She laughed at her folly. After dinner Pete and Joe Bob went for a walk. Pete lit up a rollie and they set off on a similar route Pete had done that morning. They had a kind of understanding about each other's art.

The blue sierra drove by. Connor tonight phoned in to… well he did not know where, to a faceless voice (in the military installation where all this work was based, he supposed). Those two rogues together could cause problems, they might by association make it harder for them to be regulated and at worse two psychic renegades could join together. This had never happened, MI8 had always succeeded in paranoia tactics. Divide and conquer and the like, to make them feel abnormal and ashamed. Bazza was told just to wait a street away from the hostel. Back at the military installation a man homed in on them using advanced satellite technology and watched; pointless, he told himself, and zoomed in on Bazza and Connor. They were leaning against the car smoking and watching the setting sun. Yes, sometimes their workers could become "disillusioned" with the job. And all the time he kept a check on worker movements another guy listened in on bugs put in houses by the internal security division. It was to detect any switches of sides. Unification against the land's power had to be stopped.

Meanwhile Joe Bob and Pete began their conversation.

"So I've always enjoyed life" said Joe Bob. He continued;

"I wasn't taught life, though they tried. It was always like I stared over their heads, I would see some kind of beauty and they'd always contradict it, like I think they meant it, it often made me sad. Friendships were often the same." he became confused but he needed to talk about this, he couldn't with them.

"I'd throw in some of this, this mojo and sometimes they thought it was the best but they never replied, they talked their own language and when I threw in their language the first thing they said was mine was wrong. What could I do? I withdrew and pondered my sight of beauty." There was no need for Joe Bob to pause and check for any empathy during his illustration, for Pete could react to his mind as he talked like a twin.

"Yeah man I know what you mean, the other language.

I've met guys who can speak it but it's like they are under superiors or something, they acknowledge me but it's like I have to be initiated into "the way" and I said fuck that. They watched me, they made strange shit happen, it was extreme. I lived with them and their ways but in the mind they kicked my ass."

Joe Bob stopped. They turned around and walked back to the hostel where they made coffee, then continued and said,

"A toast, fuck them!" They dinged their mugs together and both said,

"Fuck them, and happy days." Dwight entered and they chilled. The television was on and it was 9 o'clock, time for the soap opera. Pete and Joe Bob looked at each other and said,

"Chill, 'til another time." Around 10 o'clock Padraic poked his head in and said,

"Meds, people." All the residents queued at the office door. Dwight, Pete and Joe Bob hung back laughing at a Bill Hicks programme they'd seen which had taken the mick out of the none smokers. Rhona made an appearance and was at the head of the queue. Padraic didn't smoke but he could appreciate the humour.

With regards to his view on this whole rogue telepathy versus the government - he'd noticed that blue sierra and he sometimes came in to see Joe Bob. He would see him smiling; it happened a few times and it was only when he tried to return it and couldn't that he saw it as kind of "sinister." He couldn't do it, it needed control and he wondered if this issue would ever be brought to a head; would Joe Bob ever be beaten by this someone else? He didn't know, he just made sure all the residents were happy, got fed and didn't get involved in "issues."

The tablets made Pete tired but at least this resulted in healthy deep dreamy sleep. He dreamt he had lots of new friends and for a whole hour he had a happy dream, he was untouched by that state dream weaver from the other night. Then they (the friends) left him and a man came in with ripped clothes and barked like a strange dog then said,

"You've no friends, they all hate you." Pete saw them in the distance nodding their heads.

"They all hate you." Pete woke up and saw a horned devil drawn on the ceiling, it was moving about lashing its tail, it looked drawn like in a cartoon. Once again Pete was forced to say "Fuck it." The devil smiled at him. Kind of a war on two fronts, Pete reflected.

Chapter 13
A New Day and a Happy Night

Next day there was a knock on Pete's door. It was Padraic. Time for morning medication, and as it was Saturday there was a big fry-up on the go. Pete and Joe Bob had big plans for today and they looked forward to the night. After a fry-up of bacon, eggs, beans, toast, tomato, black pudding and sausage it was time for the Saturday chores. Pete and Danny set to work cleaning the kitchen. This involved mopping the floor, cleaning the oven, bleaching the surfaces and doing the breakfast dishes. The other tenants did hoovering, dusting, window cleaning as well as more mopping in the utility room.

Then they all watched an Italian football program that Ryan wanted to see. During it they played pitch and toss to see who would lose and make the teas. Dwight lost so he made them, five teas. Ryan was really into the football and he suggested they all go to see the local team play, last match of the season.

It was two miles down the road in the opposite way to the way Pete went yesterday. After a couple of hundred yards they were joined by other supporters. The atmosphere was electric. Pete even saw the consultant from the Stevens ward and he gave him a hearty wave. There were stands selling pork pies and coaches busing in fans from all over the country. They got to the ticket booth and paid the £18 and went to the north stand where Dwight, Ryan, Pete and Joe Bob sat down. An under twelve year old final was being played, the main match was due to kick off in a half hour.

Two hours later, warmed up for tonight, they were back at the hostel at the table waiting for their dinner - champ, sausages and beans. It had been an alright day. Pete couldn't remember all the players' names but he had got involved with all the singing and shouting. Pete reflected that there had been a moment, during the second half, where he had felt the whole atmosphere disappear. He felt alone among thousands of people. He worried; it wasn't Nile though he was about, doing something else. He tried to look over at his friends; they might as well have been made of wax, them being near was of little help. He looked, he saw he wasn't alone, he was with hundreds of demons. All were quiet but stood with him like the fans. Pete struggled all the more; they wanted him to stay, but gradually on the way back home he reclaimed his perception. He was back on his feet. This happened often to Pete. He didn't get scared, it was just a hardship of life he had to deal with.

At dinner Pete and Joe Bob were getting excited. Tonight was the five hour bonanza dance night with the all time greatest 'DJ Nutts' at the students' union. But that wasn't starting until 9pm. They had an hour or so before they left, so everyone apart from Danny headed out to the bar again. The barman stopped cleaning the glasses and sorted out his group of regulars.

Pete and Joe Bob left the others at 8:30pm and got the bus to the union. Its patronage had gone down hill in recent years; not so many students went any more, it was mostly full of a bad element these days. They sat at a table and watched a couple of chavs pushing low grade ecstasy for £4 a hit. The warm up DJ was playing some funky soul music. They hung back for a while, then he came on - DJ Nutts the magnificent. There were spot lights flashing red and green with the occasional strobe blasted in. The dry ice machine spread a silver smoke over the dance floor. Half the crowd danced while the others watched for now. Track after track of banging trance tracks that Pete really dug played.

At ten minutes past ten Joe Bob nodded to Pete,

"It's time to go." Both got up and danced to the bass line. Drum and bass - as old as time itself. They thumped their legs on the floor and let the rhythm take over them. They were getting inside the track which seamlessly became the next. They waved their arms and introduced a guitar sounding thing that brought in an extra dimension. They were in. The DJ's hands were on a roll, the night was taking off. It was totally infectious, people felt something was going on and the people didn't care. Someone noticed that Joe Bob and Pete were right on top of the music and they were. The music kept evolving a new dimension here and another one there, it felt good. Joe Bob was getting confident and as he flexed his hand a beat changed, when he tapped his feet differently another was added.

Not only was everyone having a top night, the DJ felt it was one of his greatest performances ever, he thought there was something mesmerizing in the crowd, they were having such a good time. Pete and Joe Bob were pretty high too. Pete joined in and became adventurous too. A few girls at the side watched and laughed as he seemingly created the music. Beautiful but enchanting.

At the end of the night they left with everyone else, sweat

dripping down their cheeks and the night's beats remaining pulsing in their very soul. People gathered outside, talking and taking in a starry night. A couple of people stared uneasily at them;

"Those guys were really into it."

"Yes we were" they laughed.

The key advisors had had them followed and upon hearing the report decided that if it had been one of their own tonight they would have been severely dealt with, but they'd been trying to deal with these two for a few years now and they always got back up, but they would keep trying to crush them. The programmers had sent back an analysis saying the best way to accomplish their aims, inflicting punishments for these two (for now they were dealt together for efficiency) was to have a go at making their future "uncomfortable." They knew just the person - funnily it was Voodoo man's father - one of their resident professors.

He felt he'd brought up his son well, he disliked bureaucracy or the rigid nature of the organization and he'd taught him this, but agreed with their cause, there had to be order. MI8 often brought him in for tough cases and he was especially good and successful at hounding individuals' futures. He scanned Pete's and Joe Bob's files and felt a vibe, that was all he needed.

As their futures were now linked the professor too decided it would be applicable to work on them together. He cracked his knuckles and bent his fingers that were double jointed, they went way back at a disconcerting angle. He lay back on a seat he'd bought specifically for the purpose of channelling others' visions, it was so comfortable. Gradually using a yoga technique he concentrated on his feet alone then worked his way, slowly, doing the rest of his body then he thought of his two assignments. He worked slowly, his head began to rock here and there in a way that encouraged his mind into a trance and soothed him. He felt like a knife and he began to viciously stab Pete and Joe Bob's vibe which had developed into two pictures in his vision. It took a comparatively long time but suddenly they fell down, flat on the ground. He'd got them when they weren't ready, they were flat on their faces.

Pete and Joe Bob were sat in the smoking room. Louise was miffed they'd got back so late and they were in trouble,

"You need to follow the rules." she cried. Back upstairs they were still high from the dancing.

"Do you feel it, Joe Bob?"

"Yeah, I feel rush. You ever done that shit before?" he asked.

"Done a few times in uni, and a couple of times on the radio, nothing like it." They sat contemplating that night's beats. Pete felt a gnawing at the back of his head and noticed that Joe Bob seemed to detect a pain as well. It was usual for Pete to get attacked sometimes, and it happened when he'd rubbed someone up the wrong way, yet it was unusual for him to share this. It made him smile, but the pain was making him irritated, then uncomfortable, then uneasy. He looked at Joe Bob and said so his mind could hear,

"Fall down in three." and they did, though they still sat in the armchairs.

The professor upon seeing them fall flew over the top of them and lifted them up as they rested their faces on the ground. He lifted them simultaneously changing their surroundings into a realm like the one Wolfie was lost in, but this one was not the same. As they got to their feet and looked around it was hot and the earth was red. It had not worked the way he wanted, they did not seem disturbed or mentally in pain which he needed to work on them further. The realm was meant to be hell, why weren't they reacting? He appeared before them and in the way of a man infuriated and under pressure of his reputation for his work assignment he exclaimed with all his might and even his soul a hatred for them, so dark a motion that the professor physically blacked out. He awoke on his comfy chair. He was shaking, he couldn't stop, he was having some sort of breakdown.

Pete and Joe Bob saw him cry out, saw his glowering face dissipate in great agony. For someone to do this, they pondered, they must have really harmed him. (The professor hadn't known about his son's association with them, nor had he seen his son recently.) This cry of death was an oath that he would give everything, it was foolish. That meant unintentionally he had turned them in on themselves as they sympathised, they had lost sight of the fact that he wanted their destruction. In a way that the devil himself would have found hard Pete and Joe Bob were drowned in their own weaknesses.

Everyone in the hostel was asleep, even Louise was having a nap on the settee.

"That was a bit mad." said Pete. Joe Bob sent a vibe of agreement in reply and he immediately sensed firstly that Pete hadn't felt it and secondly that he was no longer floating in his own consciousness, he could only detect he was a bit tired. They had lost something. With regards his usual happy mood, for some reason he just couldn't achieve the mood that let him feel easy.

Pete was watching him,

"Wait a minute," he said , kind of shocked, "I am watching you and I can't tune in, I don't know what you are thinking." No reply…

"I've been attacked before but this is serious." Pete continued. They kept trying to sort this thing out but couldn't, they went to bed after agreeing to knock it on the head tomorrow. The lone dream man again tuned into his wards and was content that they were sleeping a dreamless sleep, anyhow he'd just received a call that one of their operatives was down and they needed assistance, and that they had further developments to discuss with him, he being on the top of his field in dream weaving.

Chapter 14
This Day Stinks

Again the next day Pete was woken and again he hauled his ass out of bed. He had no sense of what the day would bring or how his friend, Joe Bob, was feeling, the only thing was he was quite hungry. He met Dwight who not knowing any better said,

"Yous were late last night, any sexy ladies, ha, ha, ha?"

"Oh yes there certainly were." Though as the reader knows he was involved in other things last night. He heard Joe Bob's door open and he hung back. He asked,

"Still the same?" - no response,

"Still the same?"

"Yep." said Joe Bob. Pete began over breakfast to get a plan together. He munched some marmalade on toast and sipped a coffee, enjoying its bitterness, not listening to Abigail, Ryan and Dwight chatting - something about a couple at the day centre getting together. Pete looked up, he tried to make eye contact with Rhona. She looked away. Joe Bob was also lost in his thoughts and although he had a slight grin as the others laughed his eyes betrayed panic. Padraic popped his head in,

"Bus here, ladies and gents." It was time for the weekly Sunday ramble, the beach today. Only Pete and Joe Bob remained. Padraic talked on the phone in the office.

"Any ideas or plans?" Pete queried.

"Might go away in time, as it happened that we are both the same that suggests an external force, no fluke, if we could get on top of that..."

"Well, that's a start but we're in the know and we've tried... We need someone on our side who is still, ah, knowing that we might have missed something, going to help."

"The only people I know, that I can think of," murmured Joe Bob, "are those cranks at the spiritualist church."

The guys spent the day relaxing and trying to take their new mentality unawares, but with little success. Pete decided he'd help Padraic with lunch - sandwiches and soup, potato and leek for today. Pete just concentrated on the preparation and Padraic noticed that Pete no longer seemed distracted, nor was he involving his good self in these distractions. He must be getting better, he thought. They continued and put the food out on the table. Padriac met Joe

Bob's eyes and was about to pull away when he remarked that there was nothing there. Strange, two at once! Maybe he'd seen the last of that blue sierra outside, he chuckled to himself.

"Wolfie, hey Wolfie Joe Bob, Wolfie, he'll sort it out if I can find him."

Joe Bob said he might as well have a go. Pete went to his room and sat on the bed, no time to spare. He closed his eyes and became mindless then, nice and calm he imagined his new situation and the misery of it and cried out,

"Wolfie, Wolfie come here." There was a gush and Voodoo man's voice cackled - a dark manic aura that he didn't have last time in the Golden Horse. Pete had run up against a brick wall, only this one was alive and trying to eat him and stop him retreating back to his bedroom, he remembered the realm that the dark skinned man said Wolfie was in and here he was back in his room, he had achieved nothing. Again he had failed to get him but on top of this he seemed to be marked in this world, one he had been able to access freely previously. He left to tell Joe Bob. Help was needed as soon as possible. They looked the spiritualist church up on the Internet; lucky for them there was a service tonight at eight o'clock. After dinner they set out, but it wouldn't be that easy.

Out through the hostel gate a blue sierra drove past, they could hear "Abba", "Dancing Queen" out of the stereo. A woman standing beside a post box approached them and smiled, as she asked them for change of a pound they both distinctly heard,

"Go home it's your birthday your life starts today."

"The bitch." Pete struggled to reply. She smiled a smile of false compassion. Pete and Joe Bob quickly strode past, saying they didn't have any coins. A car drove by and slowed, Voodoo man's father was slouched and pale in the front seat, they felt a link but did not connect it with last night's terrors. It was like someone was walking over their grave, the man, the Professor was in a lot of pain and anguish still. He didn't feel any better either. Pete stared back at the passing car but there was no recognition. It was another three miles away to the church. It was kind of eerie, it was dusk and for some reason there were few cars on the road. It was mild. They saw another person in a tracksuit jogging. He whispered

"Pete" in a way that Pete couldn't say for definite if he'd really uttered it.

"Did you hear that?" Pete said.

"Yep." said Joe Bob. Often thinking about his situation as

a lone warrior in a world of jackasses made Pete feel isolated, and he was reminded of this when the jogger passed saying his name and the jogger knew this.

It was a big operation tonight, they needed to nail these two on the head once and for all, while they made the way for the church. A person watching the whole operation from a remote satellite in space focused in; he cursed them as he saw them entering the spiritualist church.

There were a wide range of people at the church, kooky old ladies in woolly jumpers and men in blue jeans and shirts and the usual array of people who'd come with the hope of witnessing exhibitions of medium-ship. They were welcomed by a man inside who gave them a hymn book and gave them a feeling of synthetic calm. They thanked him and this time they got a reaction! There was a lot of activity in the church and they sat on cheap fold up seats and watched the meeting, they seemed to be free to send out vibes as they wanted but at the same time there was a new feeling of pressure and conformity. This could work out they both thought and felt from each other. It had seemed like a long time since they'd been attacked, even though it was only last night.

The service comprised of a grey haired woman pointing at people and telling them she was in contact with "dear departed ones." She was able to talk to the dead, she said. She was in a trance, she would take on the voices of the departed. A couple of teenagers at the back nearly pissed themselves with laughter but Pete thought it was crazy, especially doing it for people who had little skill themselves. They could get trapped in amazement from the whole thing when they went home. People like the legion Nile, Pete reflected chillingly, he still had to sort that one out; he could seek them out.

There was coffee and biscuits after and Pete and Joe Bob hung back and partook. At least half the people had stayed and it took a while to get everyone sorted with beverages. The grey haired woman was in deep conversation with a small man and both were greatly perplexed. The man kept folding his fingers, a conversation of purpose Pete concluded. He looked around and sent a vibe to a younger woman, it was Jackie. She'd heard him and sent a disapproving "hello."

"This one will do" Pete nodded to Joe Bob. They went over. Joe Bob conversed,

"Are you one of the spiritualists?"

Jackie said she was and had "done the rostrum" a couple of times on the Sunday service.

"Right, the thing is," continued Joe Bob, "me and my friend Pete here, we did not really do the whole spiritualism thing or anything but we enjoyed a life of doing as we pleased and then last night we got attacked and we kind of lost the way we had been on, you know?" She didn't.

"We kind of enjoyed a certain telepathy, much the same as you have with those ghosts, I mean Pete would occasionally talk to the odd one but me, it wasn't my thing. Anyhow we seem to have lost the knack and wondered if you could help?"

"What's the knack, of what?" She did not understand.

"You know we were psychic, we enjoyed changing atmospheres for good times, we could master and control our thoughts, build up energies then release them and bam. You know we were capable; then last night we heard a man cry out and there we were, dozy, neither of us can muster it any more so we came here."

Jackie was aware of such behaviour, aware because her guides had mentioned these, these boys they were dangerous. One of the emerging renegade psychics, and they wanted her help! She was amused at the jam they'd got themselves in.

"Look you two can't just go about in trances, working the ether to your own ends, firstly people notice (they didn't care) and secondly you need to have control, boundaries. I have my guides and the elders here, of course you're going to get attacked."

Then it struck Pete, what had happened last night was they had felt like the professor was their "kind", that he had attacked them (they could not face the fact that someone out there hated them so intentionally). Their "kind" that had got hurt, the professor had got hurt, they'd stopped psychic activity and now they were beginning to see why. After all, they had thought if he was willing to harm himself in such a way he must have had a valid point. They had arranged their psyche for interaction of their kind, a right sort, a kind they were familiar with, a side different from the one he was on, this side had drained their energies accordingly. To be on a side? Sure, they'd help people out for good…watching him Joe Bob seemed to have realised. They had emerged.

"Leave the professor to himself" he spluttered.

"We can't do anything for now."

"That seems to have done the trick, cheers Jackie, nice

one." They turned to go and dumbstruck she called to them to hold on.

"I think you two are dangerous and I don't know what I did, but I don't think you're normal, in all likelihood you will get attacked again."

"It's all right, we're just glad to have freedom" said Joe Bob, missing the point. Although they had got away the seriousness, the substance of all the man hours spent (in reality) against them had left a disturbed permanent mark on them both.

"Look, if you ever need our help give us a call." Pete let her type his number in her phone which she did as she was incredibly bewildered.

"Two renegades, loco." She shook her head, they were out the door.

Chapter 15
The Beginning of Rubbing People up the Wrong Way

On their way home it was a dark and cloudless night. The street lamps lit up the avenues of trees. Joe Bob and Pete were incredibly happy. They were totally psyched to face anything. The woman from the post box moved past them quickly with a scowl on her face, a coincidence? I think not.

"Let her witness us" they said.

"Did you get the change?" Pete laughed, she quickened her walk in reply. They arrived back at the hostel. There was a folk night on in the Golden Horse and a small crowd of people stood outside smoking. Joe Bob and Pete glanced over at them, but the crowd were oblivious to minds outside their clique, they did not sense Pete and Joe Bobs' happiness. Pete banged open the hostel gate, walked to the door and rang the bell. No one came so they rang again. Dwight opened the door.

"Louise's upstairs, there's an argument between Danny, Rhona and Abigail." Danny had called Abigail a "silly bitch" because she and Rhona wanted to watch "Come Dancing" instead of "Match of the Day." Pete followed Dwight to the smoking room. Louise was giving Danny a lecture and Abigail was crying.

"Don't dare use that language" shouted Louise. Danny left and marched out of the room and Abigail put on her programme. Louise turned her attention to the newcomers, Pete and Joe Bob.

"So where were you guys? I hope you weren't back at that bar."

"No we were at the spiritualist church" they both said.

"What were you doing there?" she asked nervously.

"Ah, just went along…" said Joe Bob.

"Yeah, we were looking for some advice" said Pete. Padraic had told her at the shift change he'd thought he'd seen the end of these two's misdemeanours, that these two had become "responsible" and "resigned" to life, but the way they were bouncing about she couldn't see what he'd been talking about. So she asked,

"What was wrong, did you both get help?" Pete gingerly made up some bullshit.

"Er yeah we feel cocooned by this whole mental health stigma and we wanted to emerge into the big wide world, you know us people in the mental health system are the last remaining social group that it's all right to prejudice?" Louise did not want to get into these types of conversations and told them she had their meds.

"What did they expect?" she asked herself.

The guys stayed up watching Abigail's programme. Dwight lost the pitch and toss again and got down to the kitchen and made teas. Louise was just closing it.

"Ah this is the life." Pete said to himself, he had a mug of tea in one hand and a roll up in the other and he didn't have to get up in the morning. Joe Bob looked at him, he was pleased to be back to his old self. After the television programme Dwight and Abigail went to bed, Ryan was already asleep, he liked to get to bed early. It was just Pete and Joe Bob. No need to talk.

"What about that man who attacked us, we're back, but is he?" Even though the man, the Professor had tried to mentally kill them Pete was still worried about him, he disliked people going through pain. Being good to your neighbour was a key attribute of Pete's spirit. Our friend Joe Bob though saw amassing good karma only as a rule for comfort and he liked being comfortable.

"Well I suppose we could help him in the dream world."

"Yeah we could help him out, yeah I like the idea."

The key advisors, Bazza's and Connor's bosses had lost one of their own. They had no ideas, short of killing these two reprobates. There had been no plans, he'd never failed. It would be bad to kill them because a lot of people saw that it was these two's right to be on their own. A lot of people admired Pete and Joe Bob on the inside from afar.

"Shit." said Nicola. "We are having the Professor helped at the minute, we don't know what went wrong, but at least last night we had them." There was a cough of agreement. They knew Pete and Joe Bob had been beaten for a while. A red faced man ,Carson stood up and with his fist banged the table, the other seven looked at him for a solution.

"We will have to get some of our dead to, ah look after them, heh, heh, it's our only way, heh, heh."

"Yes, I don't see any other answer, it will serve as an example to our people, I want these two to be vegetables." It was unanimous, the "evil two" as they called them had been gulping down their resources. The rulers had lost, give the responsibility to the dead who dictated the order in their own world, they often did favours for each other but this one would be a biggie.

Still no Wolfie, but Pete felt he was doing okay. Now both he and Joe Bob had to settle down and help this Wolfie out. In silence they each went to their own rooms and climbed into bed. They both kept the other resting in their mind and relaxed. Relaxation was the most important thing in this operation. They mulled over the day's activities and felt them subjectively. The Professor was asleep. They continued. They stood at his bed side. He groaned, he thought this was it, I am going to die within the next 24 hours. No other reaction. Pete lay beside him and with a bit of skill, beside him felt his pain, he copied the nature of his mind, Joe Bob did the same and lay beside him. They weren't noticed and he groaned nearly waking up, they calmed him and pulled him into a deeper and deeper sleep. The man who they usually met in their sleep, from afar, the official weaver of the government psychic protection force saw what they were doing and left them alone.

The simplest way; first Pete nodded, he tried to show him beauty, tried to get him to focus on it and thus forget the incident for now, to destroy the root then set to work, he was staggering forward and there was wonderment but he only fell back to the same again. At best he was no longer groaning, he had slightly forgotten the pain but it was still imprinted on his soul.

Joe Bob tried. Carefully they both continued to lie there for a bit, he was coming out of the sleep. They needed to do something, it was Joe Bob, don't fight for the state and what the state fights won't attack you. Joe Bob started and illustrated this in a dream. The Professor was walking down an avenue of roses and every time he looked, his state-developed psyche engaged, the roses began to wilt but he was wearing a fine suit and had a cheque book in his hand. When he tried to get the roses' beauty he was no longer influencing for the state and there were the most beautiful roses, yet he was now dressed in rags and carried a beggar's hat. He started to wake up, he felt poor in himself but the land he lived in was quite aesthetically spiritual. He thought to himself,

"I need nothing but I CAN GIVE, my whole life has been used to control what people have, no more, I will only give." He felt happy, incredibly happy, he doubted it for a moment but a weight had been lifted from his shoulders, Joe Bob had lifted it but he was ignorant to this fact, nor would it matter for it was a truth. No more advisor work, he had to see his son. Pete and Joe Bob drifted off to sleep, they didn't get up to congratulate one another; it had been a success and pride was dangerous. They expected a medication aided deep sleep and that they'd wake tomorrow to a new day.

Behind the scenes Nicola saluted the dead/life go-between Priest. The relationship was like a karma monetary system, one favour with either dead or alive had to be repaid and for a deed like with this one the dead had a massive favour in the bank, the rule was you couldn't refuse. One time the living had been asked to knock out a psychic cult leader who was exerting a certain amount of control in the dead's world, that had cancelled out all the debt owed and a bit. It went up and down, but this new coup would be very tricky. The dead had watched and knew who Joe Bob was, an angel just living life out, he might have provoked the realisation that everything wasn't as it seemed among people in the living; and that in turn had created a lot of work for the advisors, but that had nothing to do with the dead.

Nicola looked up. The Priest had gone and understood, and she admired his gumption.

"Well that's the evil two sorted, what about Alaska Drive…" They discussed a world they felt in control of. Their type had always been in control so there was an element of self righteousness in their work and lifestyle. The Priest passed on instructions to a ghost, who had been a ruthless person in his life, but then he'd channelled this into business deals but he no longer had any of the wealth. Business was defunct on this side but ruthlessness was not. The mission was passed onto him by the Priest. It was like this - he saw Joe Bob and Pete lying in bed, their names flashed up in the vision, then he saw them happy but they seemed to be tunnelling through life, through all the help the key advisors gave. He felt doom around the two,

"Sure." he said, he could do that. He thought of Pete and Joe Bob being in a vacuum and thus he appeared in their rooms, then he peered at them one at a time.

"Okay" he thought, this should do the trick. He grabbed them in their sleep by their necks and brought them to the military centre to the grey building with the metal roof. In their dreams they watched the eight rulers relaxed, discussing things of a great magnitude as if everything they did was of great magnitude and importance. He let the boys form their own perceptions of the scene, then he spoke clearly in the room, his voice filled the room yet the eight kept talking.

"What you two do is of no importance, do you understand?" Pete had to give him that, the way he and his new friend lived their lives was of little importance compared with the eight.

"You'll help them won't you two, no longer waste your life." It was a kind of logic, both were caught up in it, they still slept back at the hostel. The ghost encouraged them to forget they'd been dragged here and left them watching the eight. They had just finished the Alaska Drive bit of tonight's agenda. They began the next one. A serious case. A small bald man began.

"Alexander Josephs. Aspiring poet, only son of Helena and Hubert Josephs. Age 38, lives in 31 Nottingham Street in the south district. Has begun a leaflet/fly posting campaign accusing a secret group of people leading a psychic dictatorship, was reported to us by the district coordinator and witnessed doing this in the middle of the night when we assigned our satellite on him."

Pete and Joe Bob saw the gravity that Josephs was involved in.

"Hopefully we can get him to confide in one of our friends and get him sectioned in the farm, though as we have seen sectioning often is not enough." Pete and Joe Bob's reason was altered, they would get this guy for the noble advisors who continued tactics to be inflicted on Josephs. No time to lose, they left in search of him.

They found Alex. It was the early hours of Monday morning, he was still up, his room was on the top floor of a terrace house, his parents slept below. Some heavy red curtains were drawn and a lamp on top of a book case slightly lit up the dark room. He was talking to someone, on closer inspection there was noise coming from Alexander but upon listening it was an African accent and when this finished what it had to say Alexander began talking, this was definitely him (with the province's accent this time.)

They acted immediately and tuned in. The African said, in Alexander's mouth,

"I think our campaign is being infiltrated, my intelligence says the key advisors on both sides are on to us, and we've hardly got started. The city's only hope, Pete and the strange one Joe Bob are being attacked (no reaction)."

"Man, there's a lot of pressure from what you're telling me,

I am right in the middle of it."

"Just stay calm, there are a lot of people on our side, I have to go, until next time." and the African departed. Alexander Josephs still had a feeling of victory or at least a rising contentment. Pete and Joe Bob decided this must be destroyed. At first they did not act; this was not going to be gradual, it had to be done in one swoop. They watched, they were going to use their power stealthily, to get him. Josephs was going down. He lit a cigarette and opened up a tattered book of Zen sutras. He took a while to reach over and turn his lamp off, but they disregarded this. It was dark but street lights gave the curtains an orange glow.

He was not yet dreaming when Pete attacked. Joe Bob watched ready at the side. The attack was with a hatred that Pete knew to be deadly destructive for both parties. The victim felt his throat burn and tried to wake up, he could only open his eyes. Joe Bob brought fire to his spine and together he and Pete with no discrimination of danger systematically caused him pain and madness. As he cried for the pain to go they told him to accept madness instead. The madness told him to believe he was not independent of his thoughts, he was to live inside himself and never come out.

The Priest observed that the business man had proved efficient, stage one was over, Alexander was a crying wreck. Pete and Joe Bob slept the rest of the night in a sleepless slumber. Wolfie emerged at the side of Pete's bed, he was not the only ghost worrying about last night's deed, the African was also desperately worried, in a couple of hours Hubert and Helena Josephs would open their son's door and find him lost.

Chapter 16
Set Things Right

Meanwhile Wolfie woke Pete up.

"I saw what you did from afar and I came." He did not need to expand on it, it struck Pete like he'd just heard his whole family were dead. He nearly threw up at the damage. Padraic was outside, rapping his door, he could not go, he could not face him, he looked at the ceiling. It was sunny outside and it would probably be a hot day.

"Come on Pete, you have to get up, it's a bright Monday morning," then he said, "Wakey, wakey." Pete would have to get up, Padraic couldn't understand what was going on. Pete clambered through the door, his head down. He took his meds and walked sharply back into his room.

A shout from downstairs; "Breakfast!" Pete just lay there. As time passed, Wolfie tried to parley with him, he wouldn't, he had to sort this out, he just had to. There was a knock at his door. Nothing. Then,

"Pete, it's Joe Bob." Pete was out of bed, he staggered to the door. It swung open and he went back and lay down. Joe Bob sat down.

"It's horrible." Pete blurted.

"I have an idea, I was woken up by a, I don't know what, but it told me that we did it so we fix it, the only way is to approach Alexander ourselves." They both saw a shadow of evil in each other. Wolfie appeared with the African ghost.

"This is Mocto, he's Alexander's friend, he's going to guide us to Alexander and you two can sort him out" said Wolfie. This did not help Pete feel any better, not yet, he feared they wouldn't get there in time, then disaster, then the damage they'd done would be reinforced and he'd be lost in an institution, always broken, at the best.

"How does Mocto know him?"

"I am his friend, he fights the fight, we help liberate people, he helps people that those advisors hurt, the ones that caused you to attack." This was now common knowledge Pete hadn't been aware that they had been made to attack, he didn't feel any better, someone was in pain and he had to make him better, he was daunted. It had to be now. Pete threw on a pair of jeans and a shirt, grabbed a pair of sunglasses and they were ready to set out. The four of them descended the stairs and Padraic was at the bottom. He blocked their way. He could see they had purpose.

"Where are you going guys, you know, Pete, that it's the weekly house meeting early this evening?" He made eye contact with Pete, he was withdrawn, and wondered if he was on drugs but Pete bustled past with Joe Bob. They looked disturbed to him. "If this continues…" he thought, but they were gone.

"The walk is at least four miles. Let's get a bus" Pete slurred. They got one, the twenty six to east district, the stop two hundred yards from 31 Nottingham street. They approached the door, there was a few pot plants on the paved front garden. Joe Bob reached for the knocker and rapped on the door.

A woman in her seventies opened the door, she was in a dressing gown and furry slippers. She thought she had seen these boys before, something reminded her of them. It was Mocto, he was resting with Wolfie in their thoughts.

"Er, we're here to see Alex, he's not up yet is he? Do you mind if we go up? Thank you." She closed the door shut and at the top of the first flight stood Hubert. He was a bit more inquisitive.

"You know I don't think Alex's up yet, is it something important?" Mocto made him think they were from the church that Alexander went to.

"Ah he said to wake him if it was sunny…" Hubert was knocking his son's door, nothing, he pushed it open and inside he saw Alex clutching his hand round his knees crying. He wondered who these guys really were. He called down,

"Helena, something's wrong with our lad." She now came up the stairs as well.

"Listen, we are here to help" said Pete. Joe Bob used some angelic powers to calm both of them down. He began talking slowly and as he did Pete went into the bedroom. Alexander was shaking.

"I am a friend of Mocto's" he offered.

"I, I don't know him." Pete thought of Jesus, the son of God. He loved Alexander, he put an arm round his shoulder and Alexander cried but Pete looked at Mocto and could see the crying was not fighting, he had to make him fight. He didn't know what he was doing, he looked into the soul and barked like a dog. To quote an Edwardian mystic who was mostly dubious he said,

"Everybody is a star." Alexander did not get any meaning;

he was silent. Pete could hear Joe Bob talking quietly and calmly at the door.

"Everyone is as good as everyone, it's all right to be together, my thoughts are your thoughts, his thoughts my thoughts, his thoughts your thoughts, outside is nothing." Suddenly Alexander vomited. He looked up at Pete and brushed some sweat off his brow. Pete did not let him return, he gave him a spiritual hug and Alexander fell back, he saw Pete and had a glimpse of his friend Mocto, he remembered! But he was weak. He was sitting up. Pete came to a conclusion,

"I've met few people on the same fight, and we can all get a beating, it was me and my friend caused you this pain because we got a beating. They wanted us destroyed and we can't let them." Joe Bob, the two ghosts and his parents stood at the door. Alexander did not look in to his parents eyes, he'd kept his activities secret and only partly did they suspect anything but whatever it was they supported him and these two strange friends. It would be a while until he picked himself up, but he would.

Pete and Joe Bob left happy that their new friend would be keeping up the fight, they also promised to meet at the Golden Horse sometime. The sun had been imposing on the way but now it was like a kiss from the heavens. They walked the four miles home, it was so nice. They returned happy for lunch and a confused Padraic welcomed them as their morning's introverted disposition was gone.

Chapter 17
Why Not Take It Easy?

The beautiful summer day made everyone happy back at the hostel. There was talk of a barbecue tonight. Ryan and Dwight talked of going to the nearby playing fields to have a 'kick about.' Danny didn't talk about what he was doing but he wolfed down his lunch of banana sandwiches and milk and headed out, maybe he had a bird on the go Pete reflected, nice one. Padraic had invited himself along to play football with them, no one minded, he fancied himself well skilful, he'd show these guys a few things. He took the sport seriously.

They all left with a ball and some drinks. Pete, Dwight, Ryan and Padraic strode on ahead leaving Joe Bob and Abigail behind, and behind them Rhona dallied; the girls would watch and catch some rays. There were two full size pitches and some basketball courts. Pete did nets and they played every-man-for-himself. It was great, Pete and Dwight weren't too good at it but Ryan and Padraic were. Abigail and Joe Bob sat on the grass drinking the cans of 'value cola' and catching some sun, even Rhona was happy. By four o'clock they were tired. Back at the hostel the barbecue was taken out of the garden shed and set up. They all sat down in a lounge that had French windows looking into the garden. Padraic and Olivia chatted, Danny came in and Olivia stood up with a piece of file paper which she read from. It was the house meeting.

"Okay, just a few things this week. No one is to ask to go to the kitchen at night when it's closed. Previously people gathered late into the night drinking coffee and that kept other residents up. Also the night staff have brought to my notice that a few of you have been coming back late and sometimes a bit worse for wear, this has to stop, moderation people. Some of the staff have noticed," she continued, "that certain residents may be taking drugs, we will be vigilant against this and anyone found guilty of this will get a warning. (That was because of Pete and Joe Bob's fluctuating behaviour, how wrong they had got it). Lastly, in this good weather we are trying to organize some trips, any ideas?"

The cinema was mentioned and Ryan suggested some sport. The barbecue was lit and the seats were moved outside. Some cola, orange and potato salad along with plates were passed around and all was eaten by the end, including burgers and hot dogs.

Chapter 18
How can they stand outside with all that's gone on? And a new life for the Professor

The guys in the blue sierra smelt all the great barbecue food. They'd been told these two were 'end game' this morning but when they'd driven past them out walking around lunch time, Connor had sent out an attack thought that should have knocked the new them down, he was so pleased. It was thrown back at him with these guys' usual power. He'd phoned through to his boss and was answered with a string of expletives. In turn his 'super' phoned to his bosses, the rulers, and within five minutes a special meeting had been called among these key advisors.

Nicola had been making her kids lunch and had to leave them with the eldest who was only sixteen. The others made hasty goodbyes to what they'd been doing and by four o'clock this emergency meeting commenced.

"I guess tonight was going to be a celebration, the end of the 'evil two.' We have been failed by the dead and their operative, it has never happened before but our forbears when instigating this partnership made a rule that if any side failed, then the other would get returned double credit." There were coughs and mumbles of assent.

One of the more powerful yet pensive members of the group, a guy called Saul Baptiste of French origins motioned,

"We need to drive these guys into the ground, we can't let anyone get in the way, we'll cut corners, we've been let down (he remembered a witch doctor in his homeland and all his 'dopey' servants) but we will approach the Priest and demand he send one of his most dangerous, sadistic, cruel, berserk associates and that they live with these two until they either lose their minds or kill themselves. Then maybe we'll let these failures have back some of their credit."

Nobody smiled but nods of heads indicated this was the right way to get an acceptable outcome.

Nicola hated initiating the relationship between them and the dead advisors, she didn't like them or that weirdo Priest one bit. Keep them at arms' length, she thought. She said,

"You have failed, Priest." Ever since he was made aware of this he'd been in limbo, waiting to be held accountable by the living group and this silly bitch. He wouldn't hold the businessman accountable, he'd done a good job, they had had a bit of help and had proved extremely resourceful. It was the first time either group had failed in ten years, albeit they only needed each other maybe three times a year at the most.

"We are calling in our credit now. We want them destroyed and we want you to assign one of your kind to these guys 24/7 until they die or go mad in which case, you may keep them." She found the last part witty. The others found it acceptable.

"Okay."

Oaths that seem acceptable at the time they are made often turn out to be right stinkers, he decided. He left, there was nothing else to say. The key advisors would see yet more credit if he failed them this time, as they were meeting, they moved on to a couple of other items, they looked forward to a free night tonight, Carson decided football on television at the local pub, the others made other leisure arrangements.

"On to the job." the Priest thought.

There was a knock at a door. It was the Professor at the house of his son who lived in a squalid part of the west district. He had parked his sports coupe on the street outside, he felt a bit shaky leaving it there. There weren't many car owners in this area but lots of joyriders; he wanted to see his son so he disregarded this. Nobody came to the door, he should have phoned but he wanted to see Voodoo man's face when he introduced his new zeal to him. He rapped at the door, for a fifth time. The door was opened. The professor thought he looked sleepy, but as a matter of fact he was ominously deranged. He looked into his father's eyes, and said,

"Recognized." Voodoo man had been going through a lot. His kind of guy he decided was Nile. Nile had followed him from the Golden Horse when he'd met all the people from the hostel. Voodoo man thought they'd connected. His world had power but it was barren and his emotions were controlled. His reward was to be associated with a demon of such greatness.

"Oh hi Dad. Come in." His dad was one of the players in the government, if he was at his door it was to show him the boon of state power and was done so in the hope Voodoo man would see it and have some aspirations. His dad followed him into his front room. It had a sofa and an armchair with arms stained with coffee. There was an dirty ash tray on the floor and although it was relatively clean there was a smell underneath, the smell of stale tobacco, a smell of ruin. He sat down and looked at his father on the sofa. His father began to talk.

"We need to talk, it's all shit…" His dad stopped, it looked to him his son (who never really got involved in anything official) was mixed up, he looked dazed and although they could sense each other psychically he was being influenced, again it was nothing official. He carried on with the chat in the hope that something would betray itself to the Professor.

"I came here with an important change in my life." He paused. Voodoo man was interested. The whole of his life he had been waiting for his father to say this to him. He'd been a government whore and saw its policies as also being a very real spirituality. The Professor cried,

"Okay, I have been a mercenary for the people in charge doing the odd undertaking for them ever since you were young, that's over thirty years, you know this. I got a bit too hasty in the last one and lost control, I had a breakdown and then I woke up and I was well, very well, I had had an epiphany. I have now turned my back on them." He just looked at him, blank,

"Do you hear me, I've quit, I am now going to kick back, it's karma, I really believe in this shit now. I am on the good side, no more work."

Voodoo man was aware his dad was now spiritually secure.

"Look man, I am glad you got sorted, you know I've never dug those advisers. They think they're on the top, they start young and remind me of some Jesuit indoctrination, they stink, the only good thing is they left me alone, perhaps because of your influence." His father smiled and suddenly wondered if they'd keep leaving them alone, he hadn't handed in his resignation yet. Should be no problem; he did not know anyone in the business as good as him anyhow.

His son leaned back, the professor noticed in his eyes that he was in a trance. He came out of it and said,

"I am glad you called here and I see the power of change. You know I was never into your shit and I concentrated on my own, different powers and I too think I've cracked it, I have become hooked in to a powerful syndicate in the dead." He relaxed back again.

"To the dead." he ran it through in his mind, "Oh dear." his thoughts continued, the Professor was worried. He didn't have many dealings with the dead, as far as he had been told and experienced they had their own government and it was natural that they kept separate from the living. They, both worlds, were not together, there was a purpose when you were alive and when you died you well… you passed on, it had overflowed.

Voodoo man did not intend to pass on, he'd do what he wanted, he lived as he liked in the community and he had met this Nile in his own community, he was no ghost man, not yet anyhow. He looked up at Nile and he saw that he was invading his father, a circle was emanating from Voodoo man and it was beginning to expand over his father.

The professor saw his son's new power and he let it touch him. It was searching for anything willing or not to become part of the engine of Nile. He dealt with the circle, he looked into Nile and said something along the lines of -

"I could live here with you, I don't care." and he sat down in the middle and he was left away - he hadn't shown any of his power nor had he acknowledged any of Niles' power, indifferent, safe. He looked into his son; he was at rock bottom thinking he was on the top. A tear came to his eye, all his life he'd lived and had his soul on his business, a man at the top of his field, his son hadn't bothered with it and he kept his eye on his own goals and now his son was mixed up in a serious matter.

It was okay, he could look at his father for a time, he saw a geriatric businessman, he didn't see his love, he began to think what he'd do later, what were Niles' plans? His father sat there.

"What's doing tonight my boy?" He looked at his dad.

"Just taking it easy" His dad as a professor knew it was better not to react, he stood up and said

"I'll pray for you." Voodoo man had retreated and his dad walked out, the gate swing shut with a clang. His car was fine. He turned on Goldie Oldie Rock fm and drove home, he purposely refrained from any contemplation with regards his son, he didn't want to hurt either of them.

Chapter 19
Saul off Work

Saul Baptiste sat in his flat. He lived alone, he liked to play bridge to the rank 'bridge master.' But now he was alone, he was indulging in some illicit substances, some pot which he smoked after a bad day to calm himself. He picked through his vinyl collection and lifted out some hard jazz, it didn't have the usual 4/4 beat; a wave of strange notes, foot tapping. He rolled a strong one, forbidden exquisiteness. He lit it up and inhaled.

He began to think of important things. That guy, Joe Bob, a stupid name but that was its purpose, it had been one of his predecessor's ideas, when he'd been born they'd hoped he'd get teased and lose self esteem, he had, but it hadn't worked completely. He had ended up in the mental health service with nerves, those (he thought of the living angels) always cause trouble no matter what, but the organization could always try and would. Then there was Pete, where the fuck did he come from? The ones like Alexander Joseph knew what was going on but weren't exactly dangerous, they had no psychic way but this Pete was like a tiger - wild and unpredictable, and then he was righteous which made people trying to control him tricky. The only control was to make him paranoid and this used up a lot of resources and sometimes the workers asked questions about why, which wasn't good.

They needed a report from the Professor, he had failed and he wondered why the ghost people had failed too. Why not, he thought, and he smiled; he knew that Priest, he was feeling high so he whistled,

"Hey there, Priesty boy, over here." He'd better be careful, actually he was a bit high. In Africa spirits were treated with respect, he felt the people at work treated them with condescension but he wasn't in charge. If the ghost advisers ever got fed up with them it would be grave, but he knew how to stay on the winning team, anyway he could see the Priest was beginning to notice his call. So he stubbed out the spliff, half smoked.

The Priest came. Saul created a space of welcome and they looked at each other for a second. Saul had projected a grin that was aimed to create a favourable foundation, the other accepted the gesture and they began to speak.

At the minute the Priest was waiting for things to fall in

place and hadn't made a move on this most delicate matter. Saul asked who he'd put on the job and he mentioned the "businessman."

"It was a job well done, we had blackened their innocence, they weren't willing to play any more, we had..." He explained the Josephs incident.

"Yes, we were doing his file last night."

"Well that's how it was." He explained the dream weaving and them cursing the boy.

"But our intelligence says that the two approached Alex with help, help from our side and the work was rectified." Saul had a mild twinge of panic. First he felt cheated and silly.

"Are you okay?" asked the Priest. This had sealed it, the dope accelerated his paranoia. The Priest went on,

"We put out a call in our world, via less unofficial channels. If your lot want these people of influence harmed with, eh, prejudice the negative karma, it would for us be of too great damage, so at the minute the devil's people are contemplating it. We don't want a thing to do with it, this will be the third time I believe."

"Yes, one of our leading operatives failed and hasn't been answering…" If Pete and Joe Bob had shrugged off the best of the dead advisors, was the Professor okay? Had those evil two driven him to insanity, he'd phone through to their active investigation unit and bring the Professor before the eight. The Priest was backing off, he saw Saul Baptiste as a drowning jinx, whose struggles would soon be making bigger splashes. But Saul didn't want to drown in the negativity that his job had begun accumulating, he'd go to work tomorrow and try to influence them away from the planned attack. He lit up the joint and realised while he'd been talking he had still had the jazz blaring out. He went to sleep and had a troubled dream.

Chapter 20
The Answers

A dichotomy had appeared; Nile while looking at Voodoo man's father's recent karma had seen his former employer's wishes to destroy Pete,

"We can do that." Nile said, but on the other side Voodoo man's father wanted to help Pete and Joe Bob, the people who had forced a change in him. A double front was moving towards the evil two. They were unaware, they would fight when it arrived.

Alexander Josephs meanwhile was looking to develop himself, he saw the great psychic powers that he'd met this morning that were fighting for what he believed and he wanted to be one of them. His family had never been very psychic but had been relatively left alone. One day a prefect at the school had messed with him, showing off some mediocre psychic ability and immediately he began to fight. This morning was a crux. His two new acquaintances had offered him friendship and he wished to be of good help.

"Control your mind, break any programming." Mocto suggested. Mocto thought to himself,

"It's great to have him on my side but he needs to be protected. The authorities are on to him, last time could repeat itself, I am at a loss."

"I know." This was an invasion.

This could happen when you are thinking, like a breaker on a citizen band walkie talkie, best not to get annoyed, they didn't mean anything by it.

"Okay breaker." he said.

"Hi, Arthok's the name, I am keen on travelling and watching." This was already apparent. "There's a new guy in this city, stirring up quite a storm among our community, hasn't made a dent on the living though."

"Who, some nut job is he?" Often a crazy man would cause a storm in their world by new thoughts and he'd be crowded by listeners and not even realise it. In the dead world he'd be a retard.

"As a matter of fact, no." (Like he'd talk to a nut job.) "He's a Buddhist monk who has nirvana!" This was meant to impress and astound Mocto. It didn't.

"Well he has escaped Tibet and did so with the complete aim of spreading compassion to a tepid people, to help your friend." Mocto agreed with him there, western Europe was tepid, it had among the most decadent and stupid people, they were a bit happy, although not relative to the rest of the world in happiness. Of course there were exceptions. Look at Pete, Joe Bob and Alexander, but then look at all the pressure from the key advisor community and the artificial infrastructure they created that enforced and controlled the development of individuals and left others ignorant.

"Okay so where does he live?" Arthok told him he lived in the east district and that he could often be found in the 'Collins community centre' where he wasn't making much headway with the chavs of the area.

"Thanks for the tip Arthok, the other two have the compassion but they're kind of at war" he reflected.

Alex was eating dinner with his mum and dad. The way Joe Bob had left them they were not worried. They were having boiled eggs with toast soldiers. Alex had finished his egg and was now eating jam on toast. His parents were going to a bible reading and he was at a loose end which is what he wanted, to take in the events of last night and this morning. He put the dishes in the dishwasher and his parents went out of the door. He boiled some water and made a mug of coffee and plumped down in the television room's most comfortable chair to watch the news on channel four. At the back of his mind he knew he had to continue his campaign; no more leaflets though he wasn't sure how but he was going to step it up a key. He looked at Mocto and he was close, he said,

"I want you to meet someone who will strengthen you, first thing tomorrow you will go to the east district's Collins Community centre and seek out one of their volunteers, a stranger from Tibet, some kind of refugee, I have had a look and he said it would be okay."

"You mean he talks?" That was an affirmative. This fact that he was inferior with regard to psychic ability worried him and this worrying affected his concentration on the night's television. His parents got back and, feeling edgy, he had an early night. He went straight to sleep oblivious though that he and the rest were being investigated.

Chapter 21
Flies Around Shit

The team had called everyone in. There was the Priest who'd brought the businessman; the secret eight and Bazza and Connor, also Voodoo man's father, although he had to be coerced into going, he said that he no longer wanted to aid their cause and that he was experiencing grave family problems. Nicola looked forward to hearing his reasons for resignation and this "drastic family problem."

Everyone arrived. The key advisors all walked in together as they had just finished the usual quality meal that the organization always provided; they were the top dogs and bitches. Bazza and Connor sat by the side uneasy. The professor sat beside Carson twiddling his thumbs, not really giving a shit why he was there, they couldn't do anything, he was not the deviant they wanted to attack, well he didn't know how to be one. Pete would have said to use "The Holy Spirit." The Priest hovered among them, he thought they couldn't touch him, what are they going to do? Get another priest? Or was one of them hard enough? He thought not. The businessman waited for the Priest's cue, he'd been told by him what to say and what not to say.

Carson coughed and there was a hush. Bazza was sweating profusely, these people were his boss and they were players, the best way to appear was humble to them and this so-called Priest, he didn't even want to think about him. For the purpose of this conference the organization used a bit of dark technology that allowed the ghosts to be heard on the physical plain. Nicola chaired.

"Welcome everyone, fortunately we never really have to call these (collective) meetings, we usually deal quite efficiently ourselves." She smiled, making eye contact with Saul Baptiste who returned the smile with a sour grin.

"We were forced to ask the ghost government's representative, the Priest..."

"Hello." an impatient voice cackled out of a speaker in the centre of the round table.

"...to hammer the nail in the coffin of the two renegades Pete and Joe Bob, but that was only after a previous failure of the Professor here on my right. Though he did try, didn't you?"

"I don't really care."

"I told you that this is deadly serious. I already know your new views on the department as we spoke before, now what happened with the two?"

"I tried and I gave it every last ounce to defeat them, I felt terrible after it, I had a breakdown." Nicola spoke in a way that mocked the act of compassion.

"Okay, but you're better now, I mean you seem to have taken on a new life, you're a changed person, but we had you watched. We know, we were told about your "dream of revelation." It was performed on you by the evil two." The following silence was meant to indicate the statement was not rhetorical. The Professor did not even blink.

The dream had been performed in an act of altruism and somehow he saw this, the beauty, the beauty of that act took away any pride he might have felt.

"I don't care. It's the truth."

"What are you talking about," she rasped. He didn't reply. The Priest was beginning to get an insight into what these two were really like, even the businessman felt a bit insecure, yet they were stuck, stuck with the bi government pack even though it was becoming shaky. The Professor stood up, Carson had expected him to stay in the background and was looking forward to helping him into his retirement, he'd do it himself. Before the professor talked, he looked round the table, he knew the eight, he'd celebrated former conquests with fine twelve year single malt whiskeys and had eaten with them at the best of restaurants. At Christmases he'd been to drinks parties at their apartments and had met some of their families.

The Professor smiled at Nicola. He thought quickly; those two had helped him where he was now, he was fed up with these people's petty games, he was fed up dealing with some ganja fiend kid who began to think a little too freely. Or some guy who had recently turned his back on his psychic community by his own choice. He was fed up being the punisher for these people, who appointed them anyway, why all the restrictions? Where did these people get enthusiasm for instigating such tyranny? He was still smiling at Nicola. Tactfully he said,

"I have become disillusioned with the organization and I wish to retire," he went on cryptically,

"I have worked with you for over twenty years, I hope you'll leave me be." He was about to continue when Carson broke in,

"What will be your association with these guys?"

" I take it you are referring to Pete and Joe Bob? Well at the minute I don't think they are soldiers of fortune or anything." This was a lie. The Priest smiled, unseen. "But I am not going to attack them, to be honest I no longer like your set up but then I don't know any replacement, you are not exactly s,s,s,sunshine." He stuttered, aware that he might be getting himself into even more danger. Carson gave him a look that was meant to be neutral but behind it was a harmful intent. Nicola who, though, was staring into a space, had the same intent.

"Well we'll move on to the next item on the agenda;" (The Professor was still very much against it.) "the next attack on the evil two, one organized by our friends in the ghost world." The Professor got up and left by the side door. Carson sent out a vibe to the small bald man - "Last time we'll see him alive." The bald man made a note mentally to get that managed. Nicola watched his every step and pondered that he had become the sort of person who ought to stay quiet, on all fronts.

"Okay, I want you to integrate that guy, I want his retirement to be an unhappy one" she snapped at the Priest. She couldn't see the Priest and had tried to make her demand an obvious one. The Priest heard her say to herself - "You owe us." She wasn't one of the most evolved of psychics, if she had been she would have known that the Priest had heard her, it's all about control. But he regretted she was right.

"Okay, you'd better tell us what you tried, we know you tried something but they evaded you." It was Saul this time, he tried to talk with a bravado that indicated they had not been talking the previous night. He wanted the eight to seem amicable for this purpose.

"Tell us what you activated among the two." The speaker gave a static crackle.

"I put my top man on to it, a man we call the Businessman."

"Okay, we know this and we asked you to bring him along." Saul felt he was talking to nothing but the speaker box replied,

"Yes that's me, hello, I am the one known as the Businessman." Those present all concentrated on the black box on the table. "I waited until they were in a dream state and made them attack one of your other projects which they did to great effect, then," he remembered what the Priest had told him,

"the next day when they got up it looked like they'd done a most grievous deed, the boy Alexander - " (he tried to remember the name) " - Josephs was reduced to a vegetable and nobody saw our influence. That should have worked. The two Joe Bob and Pete should have retreated and, er, left the whole society behind. That is as far as I was involved." Both the spirits knew what had happened next. These two lower spirits Mocto and Wolfie had got the two to undo the deed. What could they do? To attack one of their own there had to be honest intent, you couldn't do it just to enforce the artificial workings of a dead living government deal, a fickle thing. Who that had any sense cared about that? To be caught up in workings like that would be poisoning your future actions in the ghost world.

"So you have no idea how come they seem to be perfectly well?" Saul asked, feigning ignorance. He knew they had had some help, it had been reported that Alexander was in a happy disposition as well. Like no heavy action had ever been performed.

"Let's not fuck about, what are you going to do, you are aware of the debt and that your failing increases it?" He sat down, resigned to the fact that he would not say anything during the rest of the conference, make the other seven think he was hard core; he would sneak into the background.

"Okay, I demand now that you do action." Nicola knew the oath, they all did, the covenant. A long time ago, around the time of the first printing press in the sixteenth century, a major demon had had use of the living, he wanted them to get some witches with black magic who were about as he realised that they had too much power. It would reinforce his power in this new wave among his fellow dead. It was now mental health, it was disorders of the brain. They had done well. The higher powers in his world celebrated this and the dead living government deal was born. If either didn't pay their debt then the other could let the power they achieved from the pact backfire on the one in debt, the power of the dead to be ignored and the power of the organization to dictate mass behaviour. Of course there were renegades on each side and both mounted large debts now and then but now the dead government was in quite a bit after the way the Businessman's actions seemed to have no effect.

The way the Priest saw it there was a solution, hand it to the forsaken ones in hell, they loved destruction, hell was them.

Already Nile was sniffing about, the Priest was au fait with the coincidence of Nile's paths crossing before, in the Stevens ward and with the professor and his son too. This had happened but it wasn't okayed and in Pete and Alex's case it had little power, other times people had been made to believe they were insane by such a contact. He spoke, yet it felt like he was swearing.

"We have let go of the waters, we have lifted traditional protection and allowed a nasty demon to, ah have a go." The businessman had thrown down the invitation that morning.

"That sounds great, have you used him before?" Of course they hadn't, this was a last resort, it wasn't "great" it was fantastically dangerous.

"No, but he is known to reap destruction, the business is over, we must leave." No more sound came from the speaker. They left. The eight turned their attention to the police assigned to look at the evil two. Carson turned in a sly way,

"What do you think of the two?" Bazza answered,

"Oh terrible, most deviant, I realise our work is of vital importance." You don't want to get on the wrong side of these people, he mused.

"And your partner?"

"Oh yes, most terrible." cried Connor.

"Good; when the ghost assassin starts his work you two will be of vital importance." They remembered their "special supervision training" with regards to special ops like the one gaining momentum now.

Chapter 22
Sometimes Meetings Change Your Life

The next day Alexander Josephs set out for the Collins Community in the east district. That meant he had to take a the twenty six bus to town then change to another. While he waited he was behind five others, it was about fifteen degrees Celsius and a bit overcast. Five minutes later a bus arrived and it was a twenty minute journey to the stop nearest the centre.

It was not a nice area, it was not a ghetto but there was a lot of gang graffiti and there were not many pedestrians. He came to the entrance. There was a high fence with barbed wire around the centre,

"To keep the community out." Alex laughed at the irony. He walked in and that had to be him, he was arguing with a man and dressed in traditional orange robes, bald apart from a plaited rat tail that went a quarter of the way down his back.

"Your Buddhism is a waste of time, it's all useless hocus pocus, over here we are Christian."

"Well I hope to learn all about your Christ but karma still makes how your life turns out."

"Karma, what's karma?"

"Well you'd be foolish to try and accumulate bad karma, wouldn't you?"

"Well I guess so. "Love your neighbour as yourself." That's what Christ said."

"And if you do that you accumulate good karma." The man was not sure. He wondered.

"Listen, I have to help out with the kids' club playtime, the pregnant mothers' group is upstairs, have a break." He noticed Alexander standing shyly at the door. He winked at Alex with adoration even though they had not met; such is the way of Buddha.

"Alex, greetings, I have been expecting you. I have been trying these milkshakes, how about one, there's a café on the main road, beats yak milk!" And so they walked to the café. A lot of people stared at the monk, there had not been a big eastern revival here like in capital city, eastern faith was foreign here. When he first came people gawped at him, they still did but he was used to it. They sat down and ordered milkshakes.

"So your friend, ah?"

"Mocto."

"Yes, fine ghost. He said that you have been attacked, yes I see, and it was your friends that attacked, oh the negativity, oh the menace and peril. A hired hand did it. He's failed and…" He stopped his dream.

"Oh dear, oh dear. Lucky you came, your karma has rescued you, it has brought you to me. And just in, as you say here, the nick of time. Ha ha." Alex felt comforted, yet he could see the monk's alarm.

"What's wrong, what do you mean?"

"There is a wave, a wind of terror coming your way, it will arrive tonight, I must prepare you. You will come back to my house now. I was meant to do some cleaning at the centre but that can wait." Alex asked him about his life. He never seemed to do much work in Alex's mind; he just engaged in a lot of meditation and pondered the mysteries of life. He had achieved an unnatural grasp of the mind's nature. He was very respected in his homeland for this, but he had left to support the spirituality of the west and he had started here as it seemed the most spiritually barren city he could find in Europe. A credit perhaps to the work of the eight. Mocto had been the first ghost to approach him here.

They came to the monk's house.

"By the way my name is Kelsang, how do you do?" "How do you do?" was what he'd been taught to say by his out of touch Tibetan English teacher. Inside his terraced house there was little by way of furniture, no television, and not even a radio. The front room had a woven mat and a sofa that had been left by the previous occupant. Kelsang saw comfort as decadent but all the same he had not got round to the job of moving it. Alexander sat down on the sofa, when new it had been a dark maroon, now it was flecked with black dirt. Kelsang sat on the floor.

"Now Alex my son, what do you know? Such a secretive country you live in. I understand some ghost bigwig wanted you and the renegade Pete and the angel Joe Bob out of action, all for a most pedantic reason. That your living government can't handle it." Alex did not know a lot of this, an angel?

"They failed in this and your ghost government have shirked the responsibility and on the complete liability of the living government they have sent a very nasty demon to you, that's the terror wind I referred to. And it is heading right for you, and your friends" Alex began to outline what he knew, he told him of an organization that tried to control behaviour that was highly natural, and that if you weren't on their side you were against them and they would try and run you into the ground. They had never lost until now, and now according to Kelsang they had experienced desperation and panic and had allowed a demon to be sent out in their name.

"Right, it's best I set you up for tonight before I give you any other help. These demons know they are going to hell. They don't care, yes they enjoy friendship among each other but they care little for making the world a better place. You on the other hand do care about making the world a better place, a Buddhist wants all sentient beings to be free from their worldly ties, that samsara, we call it. This is good to aim for." He looked at Alex, who was worrying. He didn't change his look, Alex kept worrying, he felt an outside feeling, he glanced up and there it was, it was the monk watching him.

"Good Alex, very good. You are beginning to see, you must separate yourself from your mind, do you understand?" He had a vague understanding. He looked at Kelsang and projected his mind -

"Yes." he wanted to say, but it came out something like,

" I experience mental pain."

"Okay, we'll start with that, you said something and thought of another." He tried to show him he really could do it -

"Love." but it came out differently as Kelsang heard,

"I rush at you and am eager." Through the practice of meditation he was not only compassionate but strongly patient, he took joy in Alex's simple mistakes, he beamed and said,

"*A word of many colours.*" It was not a word but a description of Alex and his attempt summed up in an island of feelings that Alex's mind recognized (it was a word motivated by pure compassion for Alex's mistake).

"You see there are not exact words for every feeling, for instance I'd estimate there must be a thousand different kinds of kindness and only ten words, and a million kinds of love, all can be said through the mind. Don't keep yourself bound by words you have heard, do not think that, instead say it in a way it's never been said before, with joy and pure individuality." This was some far out shit, Alex thought. Children in Tibet were taught this from an early age, though here any teaching like this was controlled by each education advisor group in each city. Of course if you were on their side; you could learn it, but underneath them, always underneath.

Alex summed up this up and again,

"*A word of many colours.*" Though this time it was Alex speaking and Kelsang hearing it. Alex had spoken, had articulated the beauty, the love had many words and had meant the thought.

"Well done." Though again this was only a variation of many "well done's" said telepathically. It was hard, few people were completely fluent in telepathy but now Alex recognized it, could differentiate, was aware, and could initiate basic prompts by way of the mind to others.

This was only the start, now he had to learn to respond to harmful influences, how to defend himself against all the evil that Nile was about to surround him with. He was ready to learn that now, he had learnt the basic principles. He smiled at Mocto and Mocto heard him.

Kelsang got some food together, the shopkeeper had recommended beans on toast, he made it, it had an orange/red coloured sauce.

"You will stay with me tonight, you are not ready, we will fight this together."

Meanwhile at the Golden Horse Pete and Joe Bob sat at the juke box pouring over the retro tracks, James Bond soundtracks and an Oasis CD. They were psyched, Wolfie and Mocto had been at them the whole afternoon, a calm wind was evident and a massive storm was on the way. They knew, all of those ghosts knew that at the least a massacre was coming and maybe even a war. Kate Bush, Wuthering Heights,

"Now there's a track." Pete said to no one in particular.

They sat down, they hadn't asked the rest of them to come, they'd just slipped out unnoticed from the hostel. A pub quiz was beginning at the bar, a crate of beer was on offer but the two just retreated to a seat in a corner. Pete said,

"So the shits on its way."

"I think it had to some day, we could only take the piss for so long." added Joe Bob. He went on,

"So where shall we fight, the hostel?"

"Yeah we'll wait till the others sleep then I'll go to your room and we'll fight together, within each other's sight." Pete had told him about the demon, Nile. Had told him about the flippant murder of the nurse back at Meadowburn at the Stevens ward and that he would get him in the name of justice. So even though it was ominous it was a kind of fate Pete often witnessed, he didn't have to seek Nile. Joe Bob was rarely bothered by such genies, he had a kind of positive jinx he didn't quite understand, they stayed away. Now though he was going to fight; he'd be with Pete, they couldn't stop him seeing their scheming deeds.

Pete began to become impatient. He thought it odd that the powers to be had given up fighting their own battles, why had they obtained this infernal mess to come after them? Pete sipped his drink; he should have got something stronger but he shunned the idea to keep his head clear but he didn't follow it through.

Joe Bob wasn't so alarmed but he was keen all the same, he had never been in a common cause like this war, he'd always been given a wide berth by everyone, people were disturbed by his aura, a strange individual, but while putting up this fight if they ran off that would be half the battle won. This was not going to happen today.

The barman watched; they weren't with their friends nor did they seem to be having the usual craic, they were talking about something of great magnitude, this worried him, he was a quiet man not actively involved in any of the movements but his knowledge always meant he was involved to an extent.

"Two pints of special." The quiz master was giving out the answers for the first round and people were queuing up at the bar.

"Live and let die" he thought, and got back to the business of pulling pints. The boys sat, they could only kill time until Nile arrived.

Chapter 23
Another Attack

Voodoo man had been asleep on his settee, a deep sleep yet his dream was a frantic one. He woke with a start, nobody was there in his front room, then he remembered and there was Nile. He wanted him to get ready as soon as possible. Nile saw himself as a promising ally for the eight rulers and Voodoo man would be his Priest, he'd get this job done then approach the eight, that other stupid Priest who asked them for help would be gone, a new age of living/spirit relations would begin with him the - dead's representative. He'd been impressed with Nile's strength but now he saw other things different from strength like a disquieting mania, but he still envied his power so he couldn't think away the pact.

"Walk to the Golden Horse" Nile told Voodoo man. It was quite a walk. He wondered what he was going to do, then he worried.

"This is your new birthday, today a new power will be born" he heard. Voodoo man looked at the street lamp and the night sky. As he walked to the bar Nile got closer in his mind. He tried to concentrate on people who he liked, but he'd been trying to build himself up too much. He could only think of his father, friends like Keith did not react to his thoughts, he wished they would. He wished he could run to his father. Nile suddenly gave Voodoo man all his attention and dwelt for a few long minutes in his mind's sight. When he flew off to look ahead he'd left Voodoo man docile.

The pub quiz was in its last round, it was food and drink.

"What animal finds truffles?" An easy one, Pete thought. It had been light when they'd arrived, now it was dark outside, the door opened and in bounded Nile and his friend. Voodoo man was marched to the bar,

"One water." said Nile.

"Your friends are over there." The bar man was beginning to become curious about these odd people, first Pete and Joe Bob slouching in the corner being secretive, now the other one who seemed to be in some kind of peculiar trance. The area the two sat in was empty, away from the quiz, the two who'd just arrived walked over and sat down beside them. Pete didn't like this guy, he'd messed Wolfie about. Wolfie did not know that Nile was in control.

"Hey man, sit down." They didn't really have the time as he'd already sat but Pete was hooked on karma, be nice to anyone. Joe Bob just watched.

Voodoo man did not know what was going on with the new living dead oath and just crept to a deserted part of his mind. He knew these guys but he did not think they could help him, nor was he really ready to be rescued.

"You are going to die." a croaky voice said to the two via Voodoo man. Only Nile spoke. Joe Bob made a spastic face and went -

"Blooooooo waaaaaaaaa boooooo deeeeeee!!!" right in his face.

"Tonight you will see your righteousness does not pay." Joe Bob was still bemused. Pete knew not to react and didn't feel like getting involved. Pete knew that Voodoo man was possessed. Joe Bob was indifferent, he was waiting for the real fight.

"Are you there, man?" Pete said.

"You especially will take great pleasure that we have a mutual friend, Mickey." The voice changed and eyes of terror flashed across the Voodoo man's face,

"It's Mickey." (He was not experienced in this reverse medium-ship, he waited for some recognition.) "Stay away, leave this life, this guy is the devil, worse…"

"Thanks for that Mickey, I am going to fuck with you later, boys me and your friend here are going to sit at that table over there and we'll be close by, all night." And that was that, the real evil two sat and held his glass of water. The quiz was over and the patrons were beginning to spread out. Voodoo man sat and the whites of his eyes showing. He was motionless most of the time, kind of frozen. But nobody bothered him, they just walked and sat around him. Nile had sent out a warning in the bar's collective consciousness and it was effective.

"That guy's used his whole power on the entire pub and he's doing it, sitting like that to put the freak in us. But you know I don't care" commented Joe Bob. Pete agreed and watched Nile and sipped at his drink for half an hour. He scrutinized him but the body was like a statue, like an alabaster Roman one with those eyes, except not in the classical dress and slouched in a seat.

Time to leave. Pete and Joe Bob got up together and pushed open the door into the night. Quickly they strode across the road. Connor and Bazza sat in their car directly outside the door of the hostel, usually they parked further down the street but not tonight. Pete looked in the sierra's window. The inside was all tobacco smoke but he met the eyes of each of them and they tried to stare him down. They'd been told to do this but the gesture was wasted as they didn't know why these two guys should be wiped out with such prejudice. That was rebellious, the thinker corrected himself.

It had been an order from the "spooky eight" as Bazza now called them. They'd been employed for a couple of years after both had a very complete career in the regular police force, Bazza in the criminal investigation department and Connor in close protection, guarding important politicians. They had counterparts in other parts of the province and they all reported eventually to members of the eight. Everything was controlled from the building in the military installation. Often people here were hired by nepotism from a caste, a secret ruling class outside the jurisdiction of equal opportunities, but this was not the case on the ground. At the start they'd been semi indoctrinated, people "on the outside" tore society apart, the outside did not need to have psychic power officially in the public mind, although it was quite natural it should be ruled, benevolently of course. It would be the eight who gave out any power and the eight were to be respected, so was the world (apart from "bums" like Pete) it was a "happy world." There were others who wished harm on the official world but not out of a positive motivation, some had even made steps to bringing them down, replacing them with an even more evil government.

Connor watched their backs go out of view as Padraic closed the front door.

"Fancy a coffee guys? Another nice summer night, eh?"

"Don't mind if I do" said Pete. Joe Bob felt a dash uneasy. Padraic's shift was at an end. Louise had just started and was drinking a tea supplemented with two 'rich tea biscuits.' When everyone was asleep she planned to get stuck into a novel with further teas during the night.

Joe Bob and Pete sat in the smoking room with their mugs, engaged in conversation with Dwight and Ryan although not with their usual heartiness. They only noticed their panic and lethargy. Pete rolled a cigarette and relaxed. What could these guys be pulling off?

"Eh Wolfie?"

"Well to put it mildly they want you dead or insane" was

the reply.

"And how are they going to do that?"

"I dunno."

"I might need you on hand tonight, Wolfie."

"No problem." Wolfie went on to tell him that Alexander Josephs was ready too, with a Buddhist monk called Kelsang.

"A monk called Kelsang, no shit." God works in mysterious ways, Pete recollected.

Medication had been given out half an hour ago. Danny was snoring loudly, Rhona had her radio on, probably asleep too. Pete got up and quietly rapped on Joe Bob's door. He entered. A dull light came in through the window from the street lights. The curtains were open. Joe Bob lit a big church style candle on the floor.

They didn't have to wait long. Nothing had been said since Pete entered. Joe Bob was sitting on his bed and Pete was on the floor against a heater. It burnt his back. Both were ready. Slowly they heard a low murmur and a life sized child materialized in the room. It kind of swaggered. Then from behind an invisible wave of a hostile nature tried to catch them unawares. They turned and looked at it. It travelled through their bodies yet they kept looking ahead. Then nothing. The candle flickered in the wind but it didn't go out. Pete looked up at Joe Bob. Pete thought to himself that he felt like he was peering over the top of a big cliff; he was slightly scared of heights. Joe Bob seemed calm, but also lost in his thoughts. He was prepared. Then a mass of voices hurtled into the bedroom and flew about all over the place, to hear them it hurt your head so Pete sat back, they didn't bother with Joe Bob. They bounced about for ten odd minutes. The outside light was blurred with all the activity, then a voice,

"We have your Alex, we've had him for ages, ha, ha, ha. We have chopped his soul in half. His parents are nice and sleepy, the ole bitch did not have long anyway." Pete knew to stay calm and composed, he didn't look round for help, the voice droned on laughing about pitiful friends, then a familiar voice spoke,

"He's right, we're right, I am part of him, a new dawn is in the making, you two will be forever associated with destruction, an epoch of hate is here, we the mighty shall survive." It was Voodoo man, who was crouched against a wall in the hostel garden, he threw a pebble at the window and hid. Nile gave him a pleasant warm feeling, then he went to make a further move on the two.

Nile set out and made everything leave the room. He sat down opposite Pete and met his gaze. He touched Pete. Pete heard him, did he believe him?

"You and me are the same. We are from hell. When I lived there I knew you, you were a great person to a great many, what are you doing here? Join me, lead a good life, you've been bullied all your life, now your enemies will be your footstool as Jesus said. Leave this loser, you don't like my ward down below there, I'll kill him. I will."

"That's it." said Wolfie. "Leave this room, take away all this shit."

"Yeah, you think he'd associate with the likes of you?" Mocto appeared. With the back of his hand Nile swung at them, they'd been ready for his hatred but had not been ready to provide Pete with an escape and so unfortunately they were barred here for the time being. After that momentary lapse Nile turned back to Pete.

"Look, I know you have friendships and a lot of people speak highly of you but it's all relative. Do you think they are thinking of you? They are asleep. You'd think they would care."

Joe Bob coughed. He listened in, wondering if Pete would turn. Nile continued the tirade;

"All you need to do is to kill yourself, then the world will be at your feet; you can hang out with me, you've been watched by thousands of our people, they all want to meet you." Pete never censored where his mind went so he thought of it, a proposal. Nile had left but he'd be back. Joe Bob said helpfully,

"I have had the same proposal before and I chose to bum about here." The guys had a laugh and when Nile came back they quietened down for him, ready for the next kick.

"I notice your friend there, Pete" he said with a kind of sneer. This warranted a glance from the two.

"You know God cast him down from the heaven, heh heh, he's the dirt on God's shoe. You being a Christian I don't know, I don't see you two as friends." Nile was suddenly in between the two, he was in the room, Pete could see Joe Bob but they had a new friend, he'd sneaked in. Nile seemed to have forgotten his past, he was amongst them. Outside Voodoo man stood beside the street sign, waiting, he was aggressive and bemused.

Nile was friendly, he had an ominous love for these guys and they did not shove him away, as a friend he began to modify them and they let him but like a wind they always blew back to where they where. The candle lit the room, it was as bright as the outside which was illuminated by street lights. There was the occasional sound of a car shooting down the road. Mostly though people were in their beds asleep, most not being altered by infernal demons.

Pete began to slip away to nether land, asleep, and Nile went with him. Again Joe Bob watched, he wasn't tired, if Pete got fucked he'd help him out. But for now he drifted off, and being mischievous himself he watched Padraic sleep. He often thought about people who weren't really friends during the quiet time of night. He never imposed though, if you didn't count watching as imposing.

Meanwhile Pete thought he would have an uneasy path to sleep but he did not, Nile gave him lots of room, it was a plethora of other things that made it uneasy. He was used to it, he kept a lot of problems to himself. His childhood associations caused him to shake, associations that had occurred when he hadn't been aware of any psychic ability, but they had. He slept. The dream was an easy one. He was engaged in pleasant feelings with a gratitude friend, Nile. They lived in this world together.

"You and me Pete, we'll love this world together." No one else was there, he heard strange Arabic music, smelt spicy food, tasted foreign teas, yet there was another side, an orthodox way the dream had. It was sunny, with little shade and desert hot. There was an accepted uniformity in this world. Then women entered and one drew out an exclusive love for him, one that he let control him, the lover, and left him with a specific way of life. It was an amicable way, though in the heat you could never feel cool, he gave the woman that he loved everything. Nile took him aside, the man who introduced him to this life - with the love of an uncle, you can do anything.

"I show you life" he said.

During this sleep he lived the shown life, it was quiet and submissive. He allowed the company of a woman to share a considerable part of his life. He did little compared to his western life, but it was hot and he needed little. Nile popped in from time to time and they drank tea together in a courtyard with a cooling fountain. It became night, the moon lit up the white washed walls of the maze of narrow streets, the sky also lit up a blue black. He went to sleep, he woke up.

Then it was a new day in this world, people were rising, farm animals sniffed about in yards but there was trouble on the way. Pete's village was going to be attacked but they were out of sight. He had woken up to the cool morning and greeted the arid land with a love, a lazy day in this strange place. He looked over and saw his wife. He smiled. The work to marry his mate was none at all. He got life looking at her. She got up and he lay utterly content, but the day beckoned him and he got up and put his hand round her hips. He pulled across a curtained door and stood outside in the busy street. A man was pulling a donkey and cart piled with corn. Pete watched him go by and minutes later he sat down with his wife for bread and honey, with tea.

It was after lunch, the stifling heat had arrived and Pete was entertaining friends with a tobacco hookah and more tea. His wife was working in the yard. Suddenly there was a distant bang, Pete ran pushing his wife out of the way, most of the street had pulled their cloth doors open and were looking up the street. They could see nothing but they could hear cries. His friends rushed past him, off to their homes, in panic. Pete grabbed a club he used to kill rabid dogs with and told his wife to stay indoors. With undeniable purpose he went towards the town square. There men with guns were herding woman and children. On the side of the street were about ten dead bodies of men with broken skulls lying in pools of blood and slivers of bone.

He sneaked away to check on his brother's house and there they were, three bandits were whipping and beating them, they couldn't see Pete though, with his fist in his mouth he wept silently. No longer would this be home, they'd be sold and the whole city burnt and ravaged for anything precious. What about his wife? He walked carefully to his own house, a bandit was at his door, he could hear his wife being raped with great force, men were cheering and she was crying and begging and shouting his name. He showed himself and he swung at the one at the door who dodged away and overpowered him. The men stopped raping his wife and surrounded him, they stamped on his head. Pete cried out screaming for his wife, he was now fully awake and he could hear Nile saying,

"There, there Pete, you're back with Nile." Joe Bob was watching him intently, he had been watching Pete's feelings but didn't know clearly what he had been lucidly dreaming about.

"I can cause that, I can annihilate your life, I can take away your life style, I will kick and scrap your friend Rhona, I will crack her neck, you can stop it, worry not, you won't be some numskull, with your destruction, I mean retirement, we'll herald a new dawn. The eight and me will be all power. What do you say? Like your wife who just got killed I will crush you."

"What about me?" asked Joe Bob inquisitively.

"You?" Nile started to snigger.

"People like you stick around no matter what" he rasped.

Pete was beginning to feel disorientated. There was Joe Bob perched on the end of his bed curiously watching and then there was this megalomaniac legion of nobodies - Nile. How could Pete settle, he had placed himself in a situation of power, now that it attracted the invasion into his privacy he felt hard done by! How unjust!

It began to rain outside and the rain pattered against the double glazing window pane that was half open. Pete stood up to try and shake it all off. He thought of Padraic and how he'd ended up in the mental health system, it had been an experience like tonight's, he hadn't been ready to give up and had been knocked back. Would he be knocked back tonight? He was conditioned against experiences whose vividness and lucidity would have driven most over the edge into insanity. And so had the playmate Joe Bob. And the crazy demon Nile. Standing up hadn't helped, he took a cushion from Joe Bob's bed and sat on the floor. This asshole was going to mess with him whether he was awake or dreaming.

For the first time he engaged Nile properly, like he'd talk to Wolfie (who should have warned him against doing such a thing). He was going to start to say something civil but his speech did not reply to his mind in the normal way, yes he heard his words but he got the ambiance of hell, a place that destroyed any time of contentment or innocent laughter. Pete didn't feel hard done by, this one was evil. He tried to retreat. He couldn't. He tried to say to Joe Bob,

"This sucks." but it came out,

"Your mother's the devil." Pete said to himself he'd have to work at this, most would be shocked at his calmness, he could still hear the rain and heard Joe Bob mumbling that he would have a long sleep after this but he knew every utterance of his own would come out twisted. If this didn't go away tomorrow he'd have to keep his mouth shut. Joe Bob heard this and laughed. Pete replied but again it came out twisted,

"You're fucking dead" Pete said. Pete had been in

situations before and knew the best way was to relax first then look at your surroundings. There was nothing here but it was a nothing on purpose, a "nothing" meant to trap one, the more you struggled the less of a reply. Pete wasn't confused, there was no nothing inside him, he was in a world, he was the world and he was back in the hostel room.

"Fucking hell." he said. Though this time he was dumb and Joe Bob heard nothing. He remembered something, yes,

"A monk called Kelsang, no shit" he had said. Alex, what about Alex? He tried to call out to Mocto but was voiceless. He stood up and grabbed a notebook and pencil and wrote,

"Call out to Mocto, Alex's African friend." Joe Bob did as asked and Mocto appeared. Mocto watched Pete wipe the sweat off his brow. Joe Bob told him Pete had lost the power of speech.

"Well things kicked off tonight, Alex went to sleep but after each hit Kelsang fought for him, not to worry, Pete's in a bad way isn't he? That Tibetan knows his stuff, a formidable ally, here I'll tell Wolfie to call." Nile suddenly appeared, he swore, he thought a dumb Pete was useless. He ran at Mocto who moved and retreated.

"Well well if it ain't Pete the mouth? How the mighty fall. I know better than to assume I've beaten Pete of the Evil Two, so what gives, Pete?" he spat. Pete felt a bit more confident now that Joe Bob and he were both totally up and about.

"You fuck dog." Pete had said it. Yet he had spoken through Joe Bob's mouth. Both Pete and Nile were confused.

"Yeah, you better believe it" Joe Bob said. Pete laughed.

"You speaking too, Pete?" Nile said in response to the laugh, but he was taken aback. The laugh had released him. Joe Bob witnessed this and he couldn't wipe the grin off his face for at least ten minutes. Nile snarled,

"You'll get yours, I was selected by the big guns of your world and my world; our world, eh? You live in "our world" don't you, do you want out or in?" Pete was again confused, what world was he in? It wasn't like he didn't care. Maybe the eight were just trying to "keep things cool", Pete thought. What was he to do, to hand himself over? But then people like the eight had never chosen him to be one of them or even helped, and this infuriated him. Those kitsch bastards, he remembered, he'd never attacked them, he'd gone about his own business, they never even approached him. He had a friend in Joe Bob, he didn't know his origin but they were best of friends. He didn't care about wayside honesty. He looked at Nile, he saw pity and ferocious power, Pete wasn't God but he thought this guy or these guys would be lost forever.

Again Nile rushed at Pete with a cloak of wickedness trailing behind him. He saw Pete in his frustration and headed towards the soul of Pete. Pete was not used to this but Nile was, he didn't use motivation to do good, therefore he didn't collect anything for his actions, he could only see the results of his tyranny as it scared his prey. But he couldn't move on without Pete destroyed. Pete wasn't even scared let alone scratched from this evil conduct and so he was attacked. He was at home. In a way Pete didn't really have a home. And so there was no history to attack. Pete detected a coldness.

He shivered and shook his head from side to side, slowly at first then quicker. He saw Nile, who clung to him, he shook then he was unaware of the shaking, his mind was in a trance, it was erupting from his temple, a lot of energy, Nile was now only clinging to bones and tissue. Pete was able to survey the situation - Joe Bob was on the bed. Pete flowed into Joe Bob and stood up. Nile did not know this, he was clinging with all his might to this other Pete.

"Look at you" Pete said through Joe Bob. Nile didn't think, Pete said it again,

"Look at you, you're demonic, you hold me, for what?"

He was holding the body with a vacant space, the more he held it the less results he felt. But when he heard Pete he turned around and, surprised, let go and then in this state was overpowered. Nile lay confused, he'd never been up against the like of these two. The candle flickered and the rain had quit. Joe Bob stood up and Pete drifted back to his own space. There was a cry outside, a terrible howl and it wasn't coming from the Golden Horse. They let Nile go and heard Voodoo man sprint off outside. Joe Bob wrapped a blanket round him and Pete got up and went to the smoking room where he lit up. Wolfie and Mocto arrived.

"They left Alex about ten minutes ago, what happened?"

"I let him go." They received the news stoically and Mocto had to restrain himself, he was quite angry.

Chapter 24
Evil Needs to Warm Up Again Before It Can Attack

The next day, actually early the next evening in the spiritualist church the 'closed circle' were meeting. Jackie was in the kitchen with another women her age sorting out coffees and gossiping about her children who were entering adolescence. At seven they stopped talking and went to the side room that the closed circle used.

There were seven there. Jackie was the youngest and least experienced, most of the others were old and saw themselves as fighters for an ignorant majority, an ignorant proletariat.

"Okay," said the leader, "We are gathered here for our Tuesday night closed circle, last week we helped that lost teenager. A drug casualty, suicide, very tragic, all the more common these days alas, yes we'll call in to him before we start tonight's business."

"Yes, Jeremiah?" he asked his guide. He had summoned his guide so many times it was like he was perched on his own shoulder. In a collective vision they witnessed the boy in question on a sunlit beach far away, watching calm waves, perfectly happy. A seagull swooped down and it became Jeremiah who the boy had met last week, square on he met him. He was looked over and disappeared, the boy had to shield his eyes from the setting sun, last week he'd been looking, puzzled, he'd been confused as to why he'd been here, he'd been looking about then this guy had come to him and said he'd solve everything. He had shown him the beach and had told him to stay away from the living. To stay at the beach and re-gather his strength.

"Yes, Jeremiah says the boy is doing wonderfully. Now Oliver here has heard something I think his guide wishes to convey."

"Yes, Heathcliffe wants everyone to tune in." The experienced ones emptied their minds and met up with Heathcliffe , Jackie took a bit longer.

It was like a dream - the seven knew each other's guides well and they met up, all the circle, and they were guided to a showing of the previous night at a hostel for mental health. It was Pete and Joe Bob's home.

"It's them." Jackie gasped to herself. No one heard. They

hovered. The two were sitting in a candle lit room with one single bed. These are the renegades Pete and Joe Bob, she thought. She wasn't sure what was meant by "renegades"; maybe they didn't have the officialdom of a closed circle, she was still confused by their last run in.

Suddenly a great engulfing darkness appeared. She was curious. Oliver said,

"These two sustained a massive attack last night, not the usual mischief, it could have been a slaying. Why? We don't know, it lasted four hours and the group of demons left with their tails between their legs." And then the group saw Voodoo man running down the street screaming. They also saw Kelsang and Alex dealing with the same darkness.

"We need to know about this, it could be of massive impact" Oliver said.

The next morning it was hot but cloudy. Pete had woken but had lain for a long time in bed. Around lunch time he got up and all the guys were in the smoking room having a laugh. Joe Bob watched the craic and nodded to Pete when he came in. Pete chuckled at Dwight who was taking the piss out of Louise the night worker.

"Yeah, really tough job. I went down last night and she said she was reading her book!" Padraic came in and they kept laughing, not taking any notice of him. He stood by the door watching them.

"They've all really come on," he thought to himself, "Dwight was extremely withdrawn when he arrived a couple of months ago." He met Dwight's eyes and smiled. Pete saw they should try and keep talking as he did not want to acknowledge that Padraic was any different here; to do so could cause him to throw a psychic smirk at them.

"So Padraic, what have you got planned today?" Pete asked.

"Well I am pleased to say that we are going to the 3D cinema tonight, about seven." Everyone was looking forward to that.

"A good job, this" Padraic thought again to himself as the tenants were all delighted. He watched Pete and Joe Bob, they seemed to be a bit tired but lucid enough. He would keep an eye on them; they seemed to have a bit more than a mental illness.

"Em, excuse me, there's soup in the kitchen. Ryan remember you're on the dishes." Everyone lumbered down the stairs leaving the television on;

"A man near the west district was attacked for no reason, the beating was savage and unprovoked, anyone with information please call the city police on …."

Voodoo man woke up, it had been a depressing night, he'd been used in that bar, he'd been left behind a wall. All this while the person he followed set upon that guy from the hospital and his weirdo mate. Nile had been even more oppressive when he had told Voodoo man to go home, he'd made his heart thump, he thought he was going to die and had screamed. Then Nile had been ominously quiet on the long walk to the squalid west district.

An old man had been walking back from the late shift at the local airport and the place was usually deserted. Voodoo man had strode towards him glad he was nearly home, to sleep, he hoped Nile would not watch him dream.

"Kill that motherfucker." They were the first words Nile had said for ages.

"Or I'll kill you." He thought of his heart attack and ran at the guy fists raised and thumped down on the man's head. The man gave a yelp and fell to the ground. He kicked him in the face and gave a final stamp on him and left the scene. He didn't look at Nile but Nile tapped him on the back and smiled at his ward.

His flat reeked of isolation, more than it usually did since his move in with the big gun. It was also cold. He did not dare spare any guilt for the last minutes, to do so would have been dangerous, him being in contact with these men.

And he woke up. Nile had not bothered him. He wondered where Nile had been, he'd ask, why not? He felt the common disorientation of getting up and his dream had been his own. It was nearly lunch time. He fancied some peanut butter on toast and a milky coffee. While the bread was in the toaster he sent out an inquisitive vibe mixed with a respect (brought about by a potential threat) for the demon Nile.

Nile had been setting up how to manage the eight, he wasn't daunted, they'd employed him and he was sticking to them, no refusal on either side, he'd sort these guys out. Then Voodoo man gave him a poke. Nobody ever poked him.

"What the fuck!" He turned and brought all the focus of the situation he was dealing with, and Nile saw this powerless moron, he was not cordial though, with spite he spat at him and saw him on fire. He pumped a bit of might into the flames and turned back.

"Prick" he said to no one in particular. Voodoo man fell on the floor and lay there for a few minutes, then he got up and picked at his toast and peanut butter. He was following this Nile and was a prospective demon himself, at the bottom. In a few years he'd work up and one day he'd be like Nile, and he'd have people as his footstool. If these two, Pete and what's his face, were in Nile's way he'd demolish them. He wasn't in the mood to visit any friends. He'd sit and wait for important instructions. He sat for a couple of hours, his dad phoned but he didn't answer.

What was Nile doing? Well after he left his disciple at home he sneaked back to the hostel with extreme stealth and was peeved to find the evil two asleep. He tried to infiltrate Pete's sleep but to no avail, it would only bring about a relapse attack. His motives were still the same and the defence was still in Pete's mind. Joe Bob was to be left alone, he was strange even to Nile. So Nile set off to the military barracks. Nobody was there, the board room was empty and the only light was from the outside street lights. He called to thc Pricst.

"Ah, you want my help?" The Priest said with an indifferent slur. Nile told him what happened, not everything but just that he'd not come up trumps.

"Well you're not getting it." He referred to help. He started to chuckle and Nile scowled. That scowl only made the Priest laugh harder, he cracked up and Nile took a swing at him. He may have been an infamous demon who had utilized hate in the living, but in the dead world use of hate was of harm, and only existed in the lower levels of which the Priest was not a part. The Priest slowly stepped out of the way of the swing.

"They'll be here at eight o'clock." he said and left Nile in the living world like a puff of smoke.

Nile had a look round the base in the distant hope of solutions or maybe some dark goings on to waste until the eight opened for business. He watched some soldier drinking a ten glass of whisky by himself, watching programme reruns on the TV with a signer for the deaf. Nile decided to get involved and made the man feel new depths of hopelessness. The man threw the bottle against the wall, smashing it. He passed out.

Nile knew what to do; he'd pay a visit to one of the eight,

yeah that chairwoman, Nicola.

She lay in her bed asleep with a smile of achievement on her face. Her husband was about the same age and equally attractive. This was good; if he wrecked her it would take the pressure off him and maybe he could blame the whole sorry business on Pete. He'd have to attack gradually with great skill, if she cried out it could wake her sleeping husband. He watched her beautiful black hair that was long, she had no make up yet her skin still had vitality, she wore black silk pyjamas and was wrapped in a dark red satin quilt. He looked down on this bedroom scene.

He thought of a blackened sensuality. She was proud not to be innocent, that kept her on top. She was of the world and was happy to be an expert in its ways, not meditating on how short a time she could be here. Entering into her sleep he took her to a world in his mind. She was proud to be psychic and respected by the faceless people she governed. In the dream Nile blinded her and left her in a life where there was nothing. It was not a choice to be in the world she was in, there was no cause or anything to champion. He sent a disguised spirit to attack her, the attack was cruel, she had no friends to ask to help, and therefore she could not grasp any relationships. She didn't like this, she paused and surveyed the situation, she had lost everything she remembered dear, she still had her family but had nothing to give them, she felt dominated. She looked at her husband, she didn't love him, he annoyed her. She could not deal with her children, she was struggling so and could not be devoted to them. She couldn't get calm, she was one of many in an unkind world. She was having a nightmare, she rolled from side to side and was sweating heavily. The alarm went off, it was seven o'clock in the morning. She gradually became aware it was a dream, but she was still fighting. Her husband put an arm round her, he didn't know to expect this change, he got up and stretched his arms. This annoyed her.

The family were all downstairs in the kitchen. The downstairs was open plan; there was no dividing wall between the sitting room and the kitchen. She put a box of cereal on the table, her husband was poaching an egg, the toaster was on. Why weren't they fighting? They were all too naïve, didn't they know? She didn't speak. Her husband would do the school run. She sat down and concentrated on nothing. That stupid man was trying to be funny, her kids liked it. She got up and left for work.

Her car roared down the main road, it was still quite dark

and it was still relatively early so not many cars passed on the road. She pulled off the main road and drove into the military instillation. It was a large place surrounded by barbed wire, it had many semi detached houses for the soldiers and their families, there were offices and then there was her building. She pulled up in front of it. She flashed her identity card to Paul, the security guard. He was never treated with any equality by these people like Nicola, he was suspicious as to what went on in this building, with these non military attaches.

She stepped into a lift and hit the button with four on it, top floor. She went past the conference room and into a cafeteria. Glad to be on her own she tried to get her head together. She slouched in a chair. Fifteen minutes passed and the small bald man who was one of the eight entered,

"Good morning Nicola, important stuff on the agenda today, eh?" Nicola looked through him and uttered a single word,

"Yes." He went about his business of reading a broad sheet newspaper, grinning about a local politician found in a compromising position, he remembered back to a project a couple of weeks ago. He pointed to the article and called to Nicola. She didn't come over; she must be thinking about the conference, she was never very sociable towards him, he wasn't her type of friend.

The bald man was still tired, but knew he'd wake up. The rest of the advisors filed into the conference room and the meeting started.

"Okay, right let's get to business, the evil two." Carson said. Everyone looked towards that black box on the circular table (the thing that allowed the ghosts to speak to them).

"Ha, good morning everybody." said Nile. Most of the eight were eager to discover what he'd achieved. Nile confessed,

"I went for him and had no help from your Priest. I recruited a man to help me, it started okay, I had them and he went ape shit and attacked one of you, yes Nicola." Everyone turned to Nicola, she said,

"Yes." in a tired way and retreated back into her mind.

"Obviously I tried to help the woman, but that meant stopping the attack I am afraid."

"Are you okay, is this true?" Saul asked her.

"Yes." Nicola stared at nothing.

"What happened?" he asked her. She didn't reply. Carson lifted a telephone and spoke quietly with purpose. A man known as a psychic medic turned up and Carson got up to meet him by the door. Nicola was not their first casualty, but was one of the most senior ones he could remember in a long time. There had been the Professor. The Priest looked on the room with interest, but he wouldn't intervene. Nile went on to recommend,

"The only way is to kill them, then I will dictate their lives, I will introduce them to a life of hell." Saul Baptist quietly observed the proceedings, there was something funny about this, he couldn't put his finger on it, he was certain that this new guy, Nile, was not to be trusted. Regarding the Priest, now he was different, what had they done bringing in this devil? He reflected that this was dangerous. They had been keen to get results and had sold out, if they'd been a bit more patient the situation could have been resolved amicably. But then it was as much his fault as he'd never questioned it either.

"Okay, so how to kill them?" Carson said without a moment's reflection. The meeting went on.

Chapter 25
The Circle is Getting Shaky

Jackie hoped that Pete and Joe Bob might return to the church. The church spirits were watching with great interest; how could these guys effect the church and Jackie especially? But Jackie had other things on her mind, she put her marriage first. When she had begun this spirit business she had spent a lot time checking in with her guide, and this disturbed her husband.

"Leo," she had said, "you don't understand, there other things out there, they watch us, you have a Franciscan monk as your 'guardian,' I can see him in my mind (from other dimensions of a sort)."

"Look, I don't care about these things I can't see, do you not see, you're too involved, you can't live on two plains, I am here, they are there, I worry, dimensions huh? You live here." She thought of struggling and trying to find or seek a way of life that would please both, yeah she could do it. Though this way just served to annoy her husband further, but she was blind to his annoyance, she tried to drag them to a joint area, maybe all three of them…he would leave her be.

Her husband left and slammed the door. He went to the local public house and got slaughtered, his friends could tell something was wrong, he told them it was the wife but he didn't go into any detail. He felt manipulated. At closing time he marched home, leaving his pals in the kebab shop. He wasn't as drunk when he got home, his wife had sat up in bed, the light was on and she was reading a romantic period novel. He pulled his clothes off and stood hoping things would resolve themselves.

"I am sorry," she cried, "no more of this ghost stuff in the house, you were right, I promise." He was naked, he got into bed and cuddled up to her.

"That's great." He couldn't have hoped for more. He fell asleep happy, and still slightly drunk.

But now with the 'Pete business' she was curious, this was big. If she did anything she'd have to careful, she hadn't brought any spirit business home since her run in with Leo, that was now forgotten. A day later she and her husband drove to a do-it-yourself warehouse shop. He was buying decking wood to make a patio, she pushed the big trolley and he loaded it. He made a couple of buys that weren't on the list - some pot plants would look nice and some solar lights for summer nights.

Leo was thinking about having a barbecue party going with his mates on his new patio,

"Ah what craic that would be," he thought. He asked the attendant's advice on varnish.

"Loads of beer, yes!"

But Jackie's mind was as usual on other things. The guys Oliver and Heathcliffe said that the boys she had met had got into something big.

"This could even have an impact on the physical world." She considered, then she thought,

"What am I talking about, I am only lowly in the circle, inexperienced…" Then back at the warehouse counter Leo told her that that was all they needed and they wheeled the trolley to the check out. He fished out a debit card from his wallet, and paid for the wood and stuff. The drive home was quiet, this was because he was thinking about the work he'd start next Saturday. But Jackie was trying to send a vibe out to her guide in this space while Leo continued thinking.

"What's happening?" said the vibe. A minute passed, she looked into the sky in her mind and eventually a quiet voice dropped down and gave her a very powerful vision, her head was thrust back into the car seat, her eyes closed. She saw Nile hurting some businesswoman while she was in bed in a house with her family. The woman got up in a kind of trance, then she was in work and there was Nile claiming it was Pete and Joe Bob that did it. They trailed the woman. She woke up,

"Just resting my eyes dear." He had been slightly suspicious when she fell back but he'd kept his eyes on the road. She made a decision influenced by a sense of justice and a bit of rebellion. These tyrant eight people never bothered her, she was not involved in anything psychic apart from the odd smile to her friends, a telepathic buzz that although beyond her control she thought kind of powerful, but this was different, these guys were being severely dealt with not for doing anything illicit, they only refused to surrender to monitoring, they never did any malicious things. She was going to approach them and tell them of the danger they were in. The eight would not bother her she thought, she allowed herself to be monitored by them and she knew she was not being given any special attention, because she had a good behaviour record. Would she tell her husband what she thought? He was too disregarded by the eight as a hard worker, at least that's what the street representative told them (most of the areas in city 29 were policed by unpaid representatives of the psychic leadership). It was late when they got home and Jackie made a chicken pasta dish which she quickly ate with Leo and left for the closed circle. She was picked up in her girlfriend's car and they were slightly late, instead of going to the kitchen for their chat they went straight to the circle room. The leader said,

"Let's start. Jeremiah and I welcome you. We've been looking in with our helpers on the case, apparently they're called Peter and Joseph. We have sent some spirit sentries to watch them."

"Excuse me," Jackie started to tell them, "It seems that the government are involved in this and they have sent the demon we saw with Heathcliffe. The attack was a failure."

"Yes we know this" the leader barked.

"Join my mind" Jackie replied. She let them into her mind, surprised, her being lowly in the circle and taking the initiative. They followed. She showed them Nile attacking a woman, then they saw the conference room and heard the voice emitting from the black box, it blamed Pete and then Nile motioned that they should kill them.

"When was this revealed to you" Oliver asked. She told him.

"So this changes things" Jackie said. Unconcerned with what he'd just witnessed Oliver said,

"Well no, I don't think it does. Although the eight went too far in sending a demonic force to these boys they have to be responsible for their own actions. We should concentrate on sending a formal complaint to the eight. Yeah, that'll get some movement, meanwhile the only thing to do is to protect them from the demon and then give them over to the regular channels." Jackie did not like this, it sucked, she wouldn't go as far as calling the leader and the elders reactionary but they always thought they knew best and were always correcting her, believing the new members could only learn from them. She wasn't drawn in on decisions of any magnitude. The rest of the meeting was spent talking about other rising members of the church, and there were reports from various spirits associated with the church, as well as how the service had gone last Sunday.

She had to keep quiet, she still championed Peter and

Joseph. She would meet them on her own, although she couldn't use official channels. She didn't have any idea how to go about this, but now Pete and Joe Bob had support neither of them knew about.

Chapter 26
A Monk in a Falling Down Community

Meanwhile at the hostel everyone had just got back from the 3D cinema, Padraic had driven them in a minibus. Even grumpy Rhona had gone, she had enjoyed it and although she did not join in on the craic on the way home she sat at the back looking out of the window with a slight grin on her face. Padraic watched her, he knew her long enough so he was pleased, this was a big thing, she was just always in such a foul mood. They got some teas on the go and Dwight, Ryan, Abigail, Joe Bob and Pete piled into the smoking room, "Police Watch" was on. They were looking for various criminals around the country, one for assault.

"Traditional crime" Pete pondered. Abigail spoke;

"This shit's disturbing me, turn it over." Pete threw over the remote. She put on some cheesey dance music on one of the free music channels. In half an hour the room was filled with tobacco smoke and they were queuing for their medication. Pete approached Joe Bob and they agreed to pay a visit to Alex. Nothing better to do, they'd maybe meet this monk.

And so after lunch the next day they got on a bus, passed the spiritualist church and to Alex's place in the south district. It was a nice day and when they got off the bus Pete was enjoying walking down the leafy streets by the nice gardens. Joe Bob lifted a brass door knocker and knocked on the door a couple of times. Mrs Josephs opened the door;

"Oh hello boys, come on in." And she stood aside as they went up the stairs to Alex's room.

"Knock, knock." Pete said as he opened the door. Alex ran towards him and grasping his hand he shook it. Smiling his said,

"How are you guys? Close one the other night, eh? But I had help." Alex was happy to have friends who engaged him and weren't afraid of warped oppressive infrastructure. Joe Bob looked around the room; when he had lived with his parents his room had never been warm like this one. He sat down, and kind of perched on the bed.

"Well let's go" said Alex after the guys had mentioned they'd like to meet Kelsang. Outside they got on another bus. Joe

Bob was quiet, he shook his knee up and down in impatience for the whole journey.

"So this guy's really cool, he works in this community centre that also does coffee and stuff." It took ages to get there, two buses. Joe Bob was more grumpy because of this, Pete chatted away to Alex. Alex had become more psychically proficient since his last meeting with Pete and Joe Bob. He now knew how to be simple but expressive in his mind. Kelsang had said that the mind was like a muscle and through meditation and teachings it would strengthen. Alex even flashed the odd psychic "hello." Pete was very happy. They arrived and Alex showed them a dilapidated building with flaked paint and an old scored sign that read "Collins Community Centre." Pete had never liked the east district, it was littered and dirty but then he didn't have any friends from this side and so had no cause to be ever there. He thought positively that some people must call it home.

"Come on in" Alex said. They followed him. They walked past a hall with table tennis tables and youths playing darts. At the back of the building was a room, and there was Kelsang and a group of primary age children. He talked in a strange accent Pete had never heard, even with all the documentaries he watched on television. But then anything strange on television was subject to censorship. He had a kind of voice that made one think.

"So children, what's thirteen times nine?" The kids didn't know.

"Well let's write it down on the board." He had not seen Alex and the boys yet he raised his hand acknowledging them while looking at the children, then he flexed his pinkie, for a quarter of a second they were face to face and it was a bit of a shock to hear him continue talking back to the kids at the same time. Pete and Joe Bob were astounded at his way. They hung back out of view and Alex said they might as well get a tea. There was a tea room with a coffee machine and tables. They sat down at one of tables. They slouched in the chairs and waited.

Five minutes later Kelsang walked in.

"Ah gentlemen." he said. There was a twinkle in his eye. Pete noticed his dark skin and Kelsang saw this, then Pete could only see his smile, he didn't mind being shown away from this curiosity, he liked this guy.

"Walk with me guys. Come to my house, please. It's not too far. Ah, you must be the strange one, Joe Bob? And you are the fighter - Pete." They reached a nondescript terraced house.

"It is here." Pete pushed the gate open, it gave a massive creak. Kelsang laughed and walked past, getting the door. The inside was quite serene. They were in the lounge. It had a Buddha statue on the windowsill and on the floor was a ruby coloured woven mat with cushions by the walls. There wasn't much else, only an incense stick holder with its spent white ash. Kelsang blew the ash away and lit a couple of fresh sticks.

"Now boys, let us get down to business as they say. You two have attracted some negative authority as have you, Alex." He paused, so Pete told Kelsang everything, about how they were made to attack Alex.

"But you helped him out. So I will try and help you."

"What can you do? Could you zap them out of the way?" Kelsang was silent. This rebuked Pete.

"Sorry; that would be bad karma" commented Pete, linking in with the whole Buddhist thing. Kelsang smiled.

"That's okay, you are correct it would be, but I am pleased you realised, few people in city 29 would have. And you my friend - " he meant Joe Bob " - I don't think you were born here." Joe Bob did not elaborate. Kelsang left it.

"And my friend Alex, you wish to learn from me, I accept; you will be my devotee." Alex sat on the floor and nodded.

"What is it you wish to teach us, sir?" Pete asked with some respect.

"Well, I see you are knowing in the living spirit. But people wish to kill you and no magic will stop them, they don't care, they will allow themselves to be hurt by the natural laws they claim to uphold. They hope no one will notice the dark practices they have adopted. They will cause themselves much harm; they think they'll retain their power. There are some things you can do. One, you can go the way you are going and fight their advances until they are defeated, maybe kill them, ha ha ha, no that's just me being funny, but you could slow things down and hope for intervention. Hard though. Yes most hard. If you see any other way?"

"They want to kill us?" murmured Pete.

"Yes, a woman will seek you out and explain, it was quite complex to divine." (Kelsang practised divination with runes he'd had handed down to him by his master in Tibet. He did not know how old they were). Pete was slightly wary about archaic eastern things. But he was cordial. Kelsang watched.

"Stay friends, I have special herb tea." He left the room.

"I don't want to die, I've spent enough time getting to where I am" said Joe Bob. Pete didn't know what he meant though it was funny to him, ironic. He reflected that it was maybe Voodoo man that would kill them, after all he was always hanging about and was in league with that treacherous spirit. Kelsang came back with a pot of the tea, it emitted green steam. It smelt of horse dung.

"Have some, have some." He pushed a cup into Pete's face, Pete thought Kelsang was enjoying his discomfort. He took it from the monk and the others got one too. As the brew went down the gullet it numbed their throats, Pete was worried it might give him permanent bad breath. Joe Bob didn't seem fazed by this exotic tea. Alex was savouring it though Pete suspected he was trying hard and maybe he'd had it before. After a full hour of tales of the Buddha Pete stood up and said, putting his mug down on the floor,

"Well guys our time with you was most profitable. Thank you Kelsang, and," he looked at Alex who was extremely chilled out, slumped on the cushion, "I want to give you my number. And you give me yours." They exchanged numbers. He did not bother getting Kelsang's as he severally doubted he'd have a phone, and on reflection Kelsang probably didn't need one.

Chapter 27
From the Bottom Looking Up

Bazza got back into the car and pulled the door closed. It was night. He hated this car, the blue sierra was seven years old, no CD player and its heating didn't function properly, it was either turned off or it was dead hot. Connor sat with a smile on his face, he was bemused. The car was meant to seem inconspicuous.

"Well some shit's going down" he said. They had not been told about that morning's meeting and it was only when they checked in at the start of the shift to collect the car that they were told they were being moved on soon. Bazza said,

"You know I really like these guys, I admire them, they know about us but they never freaked out, we've sat out here for a few weeks now so these guys must have beaten the people upstairs. (Their bosses). Eh? Ha ha ha."

"Yeah, fuck them, those pricks, they make out it's an honour for them to be on special duties, but it sucks, why should we be messing with these two? Let nature take its toll is what I say, some shit just can't be managed."

"They'll probably move us on to some drugged out prick or some backslider, someone really important and dangerous" he said sarcastically.

"You know the wife is beginning to get pissed off, she knows the work I am in and thinks that means our kids will be privileged but you know I'd prefer them to be like Pete" said Connor. Bazza sat there, then he had an idea,

"Let's go into the Golden Horse for a pint, nobody will know, what do you say?"

"Cool with me my man" said Connor. They were known by the police so they could drink and drive, their generation were not as weary about being over the limit. They'd only have a couple of jars anyhow. They left the car outside the hostel and slipped in. Bazza went to the juke box and put on "The Furies."

"Two pints of special…Thank you." Connor carried them back to their table and plonked them down on torn beer mats. The beer went down nicely and there was plenty left in the glass. Bazza lit up a cigarette and puffed the smoke out in an exaggerated way. He tapped his foot to the music. They were not known here yet the pub was happy to take anyone's business, although there was a more sinister background that noticed them, one young man from the area thought they might be the drug squad but he didn't care as he wasn't holding anything. Though he'd remember these two in future.

They began to talk about the 'craft,' their haven from work and family.

"The dinner went very well, fine whiskey." They forgot themselves, from the tyrants they worked for, to the other patrons it looked like life made them happily content, although they were still wary.

"Someday they will promote us, then we'll get to order about some other sorry sons of bitches."

"Yeah you and me, next meeting, it's not like they'd bring in people from outside, next meeting we'll drop a couple of hints." The drink was making them conversational, but it was a true reflection of their aspirations.

"Let's get up and leave." As they did so the hostel crowd walked in. Both Connor and Bazza said hello and Pete returned the greeting.

Chapter 28
Help and Rescue

Later that night in his bedroom Pete sent a vibe out to Wolfie.

"Shit man I'm glad you sent for me, you've had some of the church ghosts hanging about you. Heavies if you know what I mean. They just say they are with you on official business. When the 'other side' church gets involved with you it's ominous at the very least…."

"Well that Buddhist monk said they are going to kill me."

"Yes, well, here I might be able to help, one of the church's juniors has been asking to meet you. She claims to have information of value, and also to keep quiet as this goes against the church policy concerning you. Usually this request of hers would be completely out of the question. For a ghost to be asked to influence the mortal plain by giving answers from my world he would only have to be crazy, he would be intrinsically linked with any outcome. Because of the magnitude of the impact of changing real events a false one could bring about horror and torment for me. I worry, I am sure you know what I mean." This was pretty heavy stuff but Pete thought he got the explanation, he'd always seen that the ghosts' revelations were never yes and no answers.

"Although I have already influenced the situation and she's on her way, keep an eye out of your window, she'll be here in a couple of hours."

"What about Mocto?"

"He would have preferred Alex to learn African ways but he'll still be his friend. Shit, I have just made a grave mistake there, the church ghosts have heard us, I'll explain another time, those watchers in the car were discussing plans, they'll be called around that time by their superiors and won't see; remember Peter, two hours. These have more power than me, I'd better leave. Watch what you say, they've been sent to spy."

Pete sat quietly and mulled things over sitting on his soft mattress. He did so for ten minutes. Then with a suddenness that surprised himself he swore at the spirit church ghosts Wolfie had told him about, they were hovering around the outer rims of his consciousness trying to entice him, he had not meant to swear. They were the ones that had instigated the outburst, to make him seem a bad person. Pete immediately took responsibility and apologised to what he could not see, but this would not make them go, they would keep trying.

"So, you useless planks" he said to entice them.

"Come from your merry band of weasels?" he continued, and looked at their annoyance. This annoyance, they tried to fake it, to make an air that denied any power over them, that could be derived from the badness that this time had been tricked out of them. Pete laughed at them. They showed him their motivation and both were back at square one though Pete did not care, he just stood back.

"Go ahead."

They retreated to muster some support, they had a lot at their disposal and in forty five minutes they were back. And they spoke;

"Listen, this is the spirit police, we are here by the request of highly regarded people that are pillars of our society."

"A simple introduction" Pete laughed to himself, then,

"I do not care who you are. You big wassick." Pete watched as he said this.

"Listen my boy, the church spirits are here to help you, it seems that the government or group (I think that would be more accurate) that controls your, ah, psychic community has skipped the normal channels and sent a nasty demon towards you, we are here until they revert back to the usual channels." Pete saw a weakness in his argument, he concluded that he did not care what the eight did to him or Joe Bob. He refused to accept their help, when it was all over he would be stuck in a rut, he would be engaging in the living dead leviathan…a deal, he would have to advocate them in future, before himself. He would not.

"Stuck there for eternity." he reflected with irony. To accuse him of this badness would be weak-willed as he was making no effort to hide it.

"Why don't you f' off and take your church ghosts with you. I don't need their protection, I don't want it, they need to mind their own business, they have no right to force protection on me and to put it straight I doubt if that is their reason for being here." Pete was really getting riled, he was fed up. He mumbled,

"If they want to retain power then they have to realise that sometimes it flows away through their fingers like fine sand, to hold it can often mean to lose it. I am not going to be party to desperation." It was a sore point. He was not only referring to the eight but all the different ruling collectives he had met. There was quiet. The policeman knew not to get involved, it was easier to maintain law on his own side where perhaps their law was needed. When people like church spirits (who worked with the living) came along there were always complications.

"Time for us all to move" said the spirit police.

"If you want take your business to the eight" Pete jeered after them. And quietly he hoped they would.

Pete left his room and went across the corridor and knocked on Joe Bob's door. He told him what had gone down and both chuckled. Pete said,

"So they've gone but one of theirs is coming, wants to tell us something." Joe Bob thought about their situation, thought about when they'd sent that demon on its way a day or so ago, he was tired and with his usual discernment he said,

"Nah, you go ahead, I am chilled out and I couldn't be bothered. If it's anything heavy tell me later."

"Ok." It was just like Joe Bob to be extremely casual, yeah he was on Pete's side but he was slow to fight, it was only when it got in his hair that he was roused to do anything. Although he was a really nice guy who did well in Pete's estimation. He went back to his room to keep an eye out for whoever it was coming. And he was rewarded.

Jackie appeared and Pete was befuddled, it was the same girl who'd helped him out before. He stuck his head out of the window and made a "pssst" sound. She looked up and he mimed that he'd be right down. He crept down the stairs, avoiding the creaks. He opened the door and guided it back until the lock clicked.

"It's you? Let's walk, away from prying eyes." He meant Louise but they were also being watched. One watch was the usual Connor and Bazza, the other was a ghost sent there by Saul Baptiste. Pete kept off the main road and stood by a big hedge that bordered a Victorian detached house.

"Okay, you came to help us out once again? Ha ha. What's your name? Mine's Pete, my friend Joe Bob who you know told me to let him know what goes on, lazy that one."

"Yes hi, my name's Jackie." she looked quickly from side to side and hoped that the spirit she could see would not report her. It was Saul's friend. She went on anyway.

"That demon that attacked you, well he went and sadistically rewired some government worker who has been trying to shut you down, then at a meeting of the other ones he told them all that it was you who did it and he couldn't stop you doing it. Now they've got it into their heads that you MUST BE KILLED." The terror of Nile's fix up gave both of them a shiver. And the gravity of it also caused Saul's ghost to fly off to his living master. Pete was grateful and thanked her heartily even though at the back of his mind he felt threatened.

"Look, give me your number and if either of us hear anything we'll get together, hey I'll phone you anyway in a couple of days." He gave her a hug and they walked back to the hostel where she went on. Jackie had done her best and telling them was a bit of a weight off her shoulders.

Now to get back in without Louise knowing; he was an adult but still had to put up with this shit. He got a pebble, it hit Joe Bob's window and Pete linked a "let me in" to the sound. Joe Bob complied and was soon at the door. They sneaked up the stairs and Louise saw them but did not initiate any chastising, the guys were nice to her and not making anything of it she smiled, wondering if they'd slipped out to the Golden Horse. She returned to her book.

"They want us out of the picture" Joe Bob replied,

"Yeah that's life, what's different?"

"I mean they want to physically kill us." Joe Bob was stumped, he hadn't done anything. He could not associate the way he lead his life with anything in terms of punishment, especially one that warranted death. He was deep in thought.

"Well we have Jackie, Alex, Kelsang, Mocto and Wolfie on our side, and no one is going to bust into the hostel, they'll probably try and make it look accidental." Joe Bob was not pacified by Pete's statement.

Meanwhile Saul's ghost had checked in. Saul remembered that he'd wanted them driven into the ground but he had not realised how dastardly the unofficial route could be. So it was Nile that had made a vegetable out of Nicola. That tricky bastard. The only way to stop all this was to go back to the start. He valued Nicola as a colleague and he was going to get her back, and at the start was Voodoo man's father - the Professor. He'd call him in, surely there was some Hippocratic oath in his mentality? He knew that the murder attempt was still in planning stages so he would not call an emergency meeting of the eight, or seven as it would be.

He went on to speak on the phone, he was in his own office, this was serious.

"Hello, Professor, Saul Baptiste here, your former employer, ha ha."

"What do you want?" he said in an inoffensive way but in few words.

"The thing is that we seem to have bitten off a bit more than we can chew." He paused and the Professor did not say anything so he continued the pitch,

"Turns out that we employed a demon to get to Pete and Joe Bob, you remember them, the people who brought about your revelation? We did have a reliable ghost but he failed and we went over the top a bit, he failed too, but instead of biting the bullet he attacked with malice, he has driven Nicola over the wall; she's not well."

"I am sorry to hear that."

"Well, we had the psychic medics over and I am sorry to say that they did not work, she just deteriorated into a catatonic state. Would you help?"

"Who did it? A demon you say?" he was slightly stunned that they'd got in so much trouble since his departure. But why should he help them out?

"Yeah it was an Egyptian, really into all that evil occult type shit that his race are infamous for."

"Egyptian you say?" Was this a coincidence? His son was mixed up with a demon and it was Egyptian, he'd caught the name, Nile it was, he'd told him to go away the other night.

"Yes, Nile was his name." That was it, sure he'd help out though he would not disclose to them that his son was involved. Being back in the business he might be able to change these people and help his son, whom he loved.

"Okay send me a car over, you know where I am." Saul was relieved to have him back on side, but he was totally unaware about the whole situation. He waited. The next meeting was in a few hours, he'd have a report waiting, it was all go, he could come out of this with considerably more power. Sweet, but he'd have to deal with this Nicola situation first.

The car drove past a check point, the guard knew their importance but still gave their ids a quick glance. They drove past the headquarters that housed the conference room to a single floor clinic where Nicola was sitting up in bed staring into thin air. The driver escorted the professor to the reception. The man behind the desk greeted him with familiarity.

"Yes, glad to have you on the job, this is the worse casualty we've ever had, and it also happened to one of the toughest leaders. She can speak single words but they are more like unconscious babble. We've had all the top medics in the city here assessing her. Very sad, it brings the perils of our work home, often taken for granted." he smiled at the Professor; he wasn't aware of the fall out that the Professor had had with the eight (But the professor had a vested interest, his son who he considered to be enslaved). The professor smiled, it felt like a long time since he'd been away from the psychic community he had known well. The man walked from behind the desk and followed him down a corridor that had many doors, to the end room. The door was locked.

"I understand you did not wish for any help, good luck. There's a buzzer by the door if you need me. Good day." They had changed Nicola into a dressing gown. They hadn't allowed any visitors, her partner had been told she just needed rest.

"Hello Nicola. How are we today?" He stood in front of her (she sitting on the bed). He bent his knees and was right before her face, their eyes level. No eye contact. He snapped his fingers by her eyes, "click, click." Nothing. He sat back on a chair by a chest of drawers.

He sat in a concentrated contemplation. He did not apologise for ignoring her which she probably did not know. He was there and if she was aware it could provoke a reaction. It didn't. He watched her in a remote mood. His mind was empty, then he went and filled it to capacity in a microsecond. It filled the room with a purple aura. Then he reduced it and returned to the eye contact. No, this would not work, Nicola saw herself as complex and sophisticated. Even in her trance she still disregarded that which was not beautiful, he reflected; he never did like that bitch, but for the purpose of this he would have to keep this concealed. He went out on a wing,

"Come on now, you're a really nice person, a nice person with nice children with nice workers with a nice, ah job in a nice country. Now why do you want to be horrid when you live that life?" Still zilch. He walked over to her and hugged her.

"It was a demon who did this to you and he has got my son. That's the only real reason I took up this job. It's not a secret; I don't like you lot, I used to be one of you. A ruler in a land of head cases, ruled by head cases." While he spoke he tried to engage her mind, the easiest way was with true compassion, it was the easiest way to make her notice him and the world that had become distorted in her mind. But her pride was slowing things down and the professor knew this. Her own side were not going to be the ones to bring her back, and he doubted if she would ever be changed if he did get her back, no matter how great the revelation, or how it appeared to her, she was a power hungry maniac. How to help her?

"How to help her." he thought. He looked at her, she was just a shell. They'd changed her into pyjamas and a pink dressing gown which Nicola would have thought too girlie. The one thing that might work…

"Nicola, I think the only thing that will sort you out is to leave your life. But do not start a new one, live in the other world, drop out and look. Yeah, I'll get Pete's friend over, a regular guy." He looked up.

"Here Wolfie. Come over here." Being a fellow combatant against Nile they knew each other. He told Wolfie about the Nile connection with regard to Nicola and that she was catatonic. Wolfie looked at the room and her. Wolfie had always found this installation hard to access; it always had a business going about it that excluded him and his friends. It was a bit of a novelty and an opportunity he would relish.

"Hello Nicola, my name's Wolfie, I am a friend of the, how do you say? 'Renegade' Pete. In a round about way you ordering Pete's destruction ended up in your own." She didn't stir.

As she didn't react and her eyes were dull he approached her mind in a most quiet fashion. She didn't move, not even in her thoughts. He lay beside her, he coaxed her muscles to lay down. She lay flat. He brought her up above and she looked down, she did not recognize or acknowledge the body below. He guided her back.

Then by charity for the twisted woman he showed her a love which was very hard to do for the hag. She still did not move but love was powerful; he knew exactly where she'd like to be that minute and he brought her there.

It was a world where she could apply herself to the maximum and was rewarded each and every time, instead of tolerated, and she was always needed. He watched her, in this place. Every action she did she was helping the world and the populous were grateful, they appreciated her because of her deeds. And there she was. There was nothing in the way to stop her going back to the world; who would after her works? The balance had shifted. Yes, when she woke up she would probably go back to her ways, the metamorphosis was not true but for now she was cured

"You can stay here" said Wolfie and she actually turned and gave a very slight grin.

"That's it, she'll be okay" he said. The Professor saw her eyes had closed and left victorious. On the way to the reception he shouted over to Wolfie,

"If you or Pete or anyone ever needs me..." said the Professor.

"But I'll keep in touch." He thought it was more likely he'd need Wolfie and Pete than they'd need him though.

Chapter 29
It's All Gone (for now)

The meeting of the eight minus one began. They were all aware now of a development in the evil two case. Carson stood up;

"Well we all know of the vicious attack sustained by our Nicola, it turns out that the demon we employed failed in its dealing with Pete and for reasons I suspect that were to do with a yearning for power in our world he framed the two. It was he who initiated the attack, I don't know how we are going to deal with this. Oh, and we also need to thank our former operative - The Professor. Saul, would you like to elaborate?"

Saul calmly looked at everyone around the table and then rose. He paused then spoke;

"Well, our own people failed in the reviving, and I had to beseech the Professor for his help, and after a chat I am glad to say he obliged. He did the business earlier and has left the installation. I am sure we are all glad that Nicola will be back in our ranks soon, she is still recuperating and in recovery in our own medical centre. And…"

"Thank you Saul" Carson interrupted. But Saul was not finished;

"I think it prudent that we discuss what to do with the two and the demon Nile."

"Well yes, I was getting to that" Carson commented. Already in the room there was a sly struggle for power (created since Nicola had vacated). Curtis, a fat bald man who had a distinct rationality stood up and said,

"We should wait until Nicola returns, and we should revive our contact with the Priest. If we had not been so, shall I say brash, this would not have happened in the first place." He tapped his fist lightly on the table. The other five murmured words of agreement. Saul sat back, but Carson was a bit displeased and he showed this with a slight scowl on his face.

Suddenly there was static from the black box, it worked with crystals the eight did not understand. Some government bureau that specialised in dark technology had installed it. It was strange in that it didn't need any apparent power source. It crackled.

"You cretinous lumps of shit, you aren't getting rid of me." There was a silence and crackling. Carson's bum cheeks were clenched together, he didn't know what to do.

"Do you hear me?" the box sneered. Carson wished Nicola had been there, with her fiery tongue he had no doubt she would have rebuked him, but then she had come out the worse in their last meeting.

"You can't get rid of me, you employed me with an oath. We're a team. I went to the lady and if any of you cross me you'll get the same." The council were not going to bow to him. Each blushed, trying to wish that another one of their council would stand up to Nile any minute. It was not happening.

Saul tried the Priest. The Priest acknowledged him with a smile but kept a distance. By this gesture he was telling Saul that he liked him but was not going to get involved with his work again. Saul sunk back. One of the eight, a sallow looking man called Jake with grey hair and a tweed suit stood up;

"Look if we can not get rid of you I would rather dissolve the whole organization. You will not hold us to ransom. Do I make myself clear?"

"Come now my friends, let's be friends, let's have none of this" said the demon. The group was about to be engaged in a battle, but not to preserve the so called greater good but to preserve a livelihood. They did not know if they'd succeed. This would be the most shrewd undertaking the council had ever attempted.

"This would affect their own futures rather than some poor upstarts and free spirits" a passing spirit noticed.

Saul saw this as advantageous, he would sit back and hopefully come out the best. He'd talk to the Priest when he got home. The box was ranting, they all got up and left the conference.

"Who's going to give out the orders now, what are we going to do?" Carson was worrying.

"Well I am sure that Nile has infiltrated all areas of the organization and there's no point pressurising him with our ghosts. We can only go home with our tails between our legs." Saul decided to go and see Nicola. He left Carson by the car park and strolled down to the medical centre at the other end of the installation. He nodded to the man at reception and walked past, up to the last room in the corridor and knocked. The door was now unlocked.

Nicola was sitting up with a duvet wrapped around her.

"I had the most wonderful dream." Saul smiled. He wondered if his news would be of detrimental effect.

"I have to tell you a few things." He told her that the attack she suffered was by Nile and that he'd both failed then framed Pete. She took the news well, asking him what the plan was now.

"Er the thing is we can't get rid of him, he's taken charge of us so we've had to dissolve our team for the time being." She did not reply, but she was philosophical. She ran her fingers through her long black hair and said,

"Well I think I'll go home for now, see my family. Without us the organization is dead, it is of no effect. It is now up to the psychic community to govern themselves." Saul was surprised, the incident had changed her, she was no longer the power hungry bitch he had worked with all this time.

He did not tell her of the plan he had to go underground, he'd been toying with the idea for a while and now there was an opening. On the way home he detected Nile in his car, he was trying to control Saul. But Saul didn't panic, he just drove his car and thought of what he'd have for dinner.

Chapter 30
The New Provisional Circle

Meanwhile as power was leaking from the eight the closed circle was welcoming it. There was a certain electricity in the back room of the church.

"The power is ours. Our guides have made known that the government has failed. The dark demon we saw attack Peter and Joseph has taken charge of the eight, and the eight have jumped ship. To escape a catastrophe it is now up to us to monitor any negative goings on. We must also put an end to the demon Nile and return things to normal."

Jackie began to worry; the church was a church, it was not some militia. And she was friends with Pete. Yes, she didn't like the demon, so maybe she'd concentrate on that side of things. As for returning power to the eight, there would have to be a big change, and were they going to approach the eight and make them aware of this government of clerics?

"Yes, we'll ask those sentry ghosts to keep a closer eye on Peter and Joseph Robert and Alexander and to keep an ear out for things and report." One of the circle was thinking along the same lines as Jackie, it was her coffee friend.

"We don't have any of the resources that the government had, we'll never have power, we will not be able to control renegade activity." The main man, the top elder, the one whose guide Jeremiah we have met, Eugene, stood up and said,

"But this is the dream that we could rule this land in an enlightened way." Others agreed but a couple of people didn't, one of them an elder who had a more charitable nature, who Jackie knew as Mary spoke;

"I think we should continue to help people in trouble but I don't think we should try and rule, just," she repeated herself, "try and help people." A couple of the other elders coughed and disagreement was beginning to grow in the room. Jackie put forward her opinion;

"I think we should try and help Pete and Joe Bob." Oliver was suddenly suspicious and Heathcliffe the spirit was prodding her.

"Why do you call them that? The guides said they were called Peter and Joseph." Eugene nodded to Jeremiah and Jackie blurted out,

"Yes, I know them and they're good. I made them aware of a threat, I saw that their lives were at risk."

"You should have gone through the circle, you know the rules, no operating outside the circle. When cases do happen you approach me, even over the phone would have done, you have made a major mistake." He stopped expecting an apology. After ten or so seconds there was no apology.

"This is bad, you have broken the rule and you must leave." Eugene was speaking. There was a hint of sadness in his voice but also a rigidity. She got up, and out of the other twelve in the circle three others rose and followed. Mary was among them.

"Banished, you lot are banished we don't want you back." They left the aspirant new organization. When they got outside Jackie told them to follow her home, as what they did now was of great importance and a plan was needed for what to do next.

While these events were going on at the council of the eight and the closed circle Pete sat happily in the hostel. The sunny weather they'd been experiencing had ceased and it was raining heavily. In the smoking room he watched the raindrops scurrying down the window pane. Dwight walked in and they played pitch and toss for teas. This time Abigail lost. That was a tea for Pete and Joe Bob and coffees for Ryan, Dwight and herself. She descended the stairs and went past the office. Padraic poked his head out, he was talking to another worker called Shelia. They were discussing Pete, he had settled in well but it would soon be time for him to move out. They thought a private landlord would be best, as for the others, they could stay a bit longer. Dwight needed more time, he had only just emerged from a period of depression and extreme psychosis and after his time at the hostel he would move to longer term supported housing, although Pete would always keep contact with him and the others. A few minutes later everyone was sipping their hot beverages.

A crumby American chat show was on the television, the episode was called "I can't sleep with my fat wife." Everyone was talking over it except Abigail who was paying particular attention to it, she could really sympathise with the women although she had never had a problem with weight. Padraic climbed up the stairs and appeared at the doorway.

"Pete, if we could talk to you some time, and it's your turn tonight to prepare dinner." He pointed at Joe Bob. They were in no rush, it was still about four o'clock. Pete was enjoying a tobacco roll up. He felt good. His phone went,

"Hello."

"Hi, it's Alex here, can you speak?" Pete got up and went to his room.

"Go ahead."

"It seems the whole eight has come crashing down. Mocto was having a sniff around and got into their conference room. All the ghosts have deserted them, Nile tried to take control and they could not get rid of him." Alex was getting very excited, after all it was them that attacked him and he'd also had to put up with being watched ever since he'd decided to go it alone and screw the hierarchy. But Pete was cautious, there were often massive changes in the system and many times he had felt victory only for it to be gone in an instant, replaced by something else. Pete would just carry on as usual. He was never going to try and take over. His friend Joe Bob was the same, anything for an easy life. They weren't bad, they'd just been absent the day everyone was told about the rules.

"So you got any plans, Alex?"

"Yeah, me and Kelsang are going to recruit, get a power base sorted, peace warriors. Start off an active creed."

"Well be careful, as well as Nile there will be others and they might not take kindly to you, but then you have Kelsang, it should be okay, me and Joe Bob are taking it easy, we'll throw the odd card your way."

"No bother." Alex would have liked them on board but he still admired them, they'd helped him out, they'd called round personally and he'd always remember that. And so he made plans which excluded Pete and Joe Bob. Alex was confident now, for so long everything around him had tried to say he was alone, now he'd met Pete he was sure there were many other people out there, waiting.

Pete walked back to the smoking room, he slumped down in a comfy seat and continued with the business of taking it easy. Joe Bob flashed him a vibe that said,

"Any problem?" Pete flashed back a vibe that showed contentment. He relaxed. Wolfie came in his sphere, he'd been checking for danger again but had found nothing so he was at a lose end and knew Pete was always pleased to see him. Wolfie knew the score with the origin of Joe Bob, he and practically everyone he knew knew about the fall of this Ephraim, not that it would impact on him but it was still interesting.

Pete showed him his conversation with Alex and Wolfie zoomed off to check things out. Joe Bob left to make dinner. Pete followed him down and sat on the work top while Joe Bob cooked. Joe Bob lifted out some chicken from the fridge that he'd had marinating in a jerk mix. It did not take long to make, he put some paprika, garlic and thyme in salad cream for a great sauce. Sweet.

After dinner which everyone apart from Danny said was great, Pete popped into the office to hear what Padraic wanted. Even Padraic felt the change in the air but didn't associate it with anything. He looked up and brought Pete in, Olivia was there too. They both had mugs of coffee.

"Ah, take a seat Pete." He smiled and didn't get round to the point. He asked Pete about how long he'd been playing the guitar which they both did, then he said how pleased he was with Pete settling in, that Pete had proved he was very capable with cooking and keeping his room tidy, then he said,

"So I think you should move to your own housing, we'll still give you support of course and we'll help you find your place." Pete was used to losing the status quo and to changes in his routine, he could set up house anywhere, it didn't bother him.

"Okay" said Pete.

"Do you have any idea which district you'd like to move to?" Pete thought about this; best move somewhere that had shops and was near the city centre. The south had the nicest houses but did not have much else, although he did like the Golden Horse. Then in the east was the community centre and Kelsang, the housing was only all right and had a lot of ethnic families living there. The west was poor but there were more outsiders there, people who did not bother with the state, although they could be equally dangerous; Voodoo man lived there but Pete did not know this. Then there was the north district, Pete had never been up there much, this was where the military base was and Pete assumed that that was where the government people lived. All the areas were mixed in with people who were ignorant of any extrasensory activity. Often the fate of somebody who all their life never noticed these psychic goings on was to be married to psychic people who wanted to be in control, the dominant partner. It meant that they were unknowingly enslaved by their spouse, manipulated, they would not see themselves being controlled, they could not see defence, especially against those that "loved" them. Sometimes even their own psychic children would turn on father or mother, often the only way out would be suicide. If Pete was fighting against anything it was such horrible goings on.

"Yeah, I'd like to move to the west area." Padraic raised his eyebrows and thought of the blue sierra. It would be harder to monitor Pete in that area, ah well, it was nothing to do with him.

"Okay, I'll get the appropriate forms and get things moving." Pete went back upstairs and told the others that he would be leaving soon. Joe Bob was quiet while the rest thought of their own stay and how Pete had been a true friend and shown them a good time. Joe Bob had settled down when he had met Pete, two like minds, one who admitted to certain activity. Pete was not some watcher the like of which had tried to befriend him in the past. Having the news that he'd be without Pete he slouched into the chair and was quiet in the room. Pete looked over and showed him a happy face. Joe Bob put it away.

"You know you can come with me if you want, we can move in together." Joe Bob looked up, he noticed everyone and gave a wide smile that revealed a mouth full of white teeth.

"Okay, I will go." This would really shove his controllers. For the first time he was moving away, away from prying researchers. They could not stop him without putting all their cards on the table and they wouldn't do that. Pete decided to go out for a walk and in his solitude he'd seek out a dream of what was really happening. He stood up and Joe Bob knew to leave him alone.

Out of the door he strolled. He had to go beyond Wolfie and Mocto. He crossed an ether, a crossroads of other world activity. He watched. Afar off Nile was working, but he had his back turned and was paying little attention to this place or its incidents. Pete wasn't in the mood to attack or apply his senses. He looked at the eight. It wasn't very good, apart from Nicola who had mellowed for now, he saw her ways and smiled to himself, she could only be of good effect to the eight now. Then there was Saul, Pete didn't know him but he saw he was gathering in his previous actions like he was going to make a move. The others could not entangle themselves from the demon Nile, they didn't know where to go but they didn't want to be under him. Their minds were hardening like melted wax and their souls needed their minds to get about.

Nile was working, he had snatched the council and was

actually trying to forge some crazy empire, to make a pass where his friends could enter the living and influence society. It was worrying but Pete trusted there were people like himself that would put a stop to it. He looked at Voodoo man; he was suspiciously hard to find. His father was having the same problem with regard to that. Lastly he checked out Jackie, he expected to see her in the closed circle but it was like she'd never been there, they were going about their business. The circle seemed a bit smaller. He felt a pang of distress but it got a reply that gave Pete a pleasant surprise, he saw Jackie, eye to eye the head of a team doing some brave works. Pete had walked a couple of miles, he turned back, it was drizzling and his jumper was damp.

Chapter 31
Mummy I Killed My Dog, a Time To Go Undercover

The Professor paced up and down. He'd had no word from Saul but had had an email from Nicola thanking him but saying that it would be a while until she was up and about again. Nicola was unaware of the developments, she thought she'd be getting up soon and going back to the council with added zeal. She trusted they would do fine without her for now, she wanted to become friendly with everyone and transform the way they all worked.

But the Professor was worried, Saul hadn't told him about the frame but Wolfie had filled in all the blanks, would Saul ask him for more help? He and Saul had talked about Nile at the clinic and that is why he'd helped, his son was in the same position. His son had disappeared, he wouldn't answer the phone or open the door, that was if he was in at all. The curtains were drawn. A neighbour had walked past but he had not seen him either; someone must have seen him, must have at least seen him buying food. He kept pacing to and fro. He was in his house near the telephone. It was the only place where he might get any closure. He could only wait.

He did, he waited for six hours. Nothing. He was at his wits' end. He would approach Pete and Joe Bob. They were outside his usual sphere and if officials saw him associating with them he could be in a bit of trouble but it was nothing he could not handle. Now was the time; he got up and drove to the hostel, he knew where they lived, they'd sent people there before and also he'd been briefed for background on the attack. He lived in north district but he did not like it and was going to move, it was all status there and recently he had learnt that status was not everything; at one time he thought it was. He pulled up outside, it was night and as luck would have it there was Pete walking down the street. He wound down the window and called him over. He sent out a vibe of humbleness and introduction.

"Would you get in, I have come here on a most important matter. I desire your help, I am in complete distress." Pete got in and he gave a quick look round, nobody, not even that blue sierra that Pete thought must belong to a neighbour was there. They sped off. The Professor drove down the main road to the outskirts. They drove further and he pulled into a country lane. He turned to Pete and tears swelled up in his eyes and he brushed them away with his hand. He spoke, it was hard, there was a lump in his throat, he had to fight against his distress to make him self clear.

"My son, he is with the ghost Nile." This seriousness hit Pete, then he began to realise, realise that his son was Voodoo man.

"What do you want me to do?" Although Pete was not asking him, it was rhetorical. Half an hour ago Pete had seen the father looking, he'd looked and nothing.

"You know Nile attacked a senior worker and blamed you for the attack?"

"I do." He looked about, at Pete, desperation was beginning to creep into him.

"Did Wolfie tell you about my help of Nicola?"

"Yes." Pete started to ponder, this guy had helped, he'd shown compassion, first he'd left a job that had put him in positions where he did iniquitous acts, and he had helped Nicola.

"Okay," said Pete, "I can do business with you." They discussed things but they both came to the conclusion that they had to deal with Nile and that when he fell they could bring back some kind of order. The eight had better learn from this.

"Well how do we get him?" The Professor said with regards to Nile.

"Well, who is he would be a good place to start." They put their heads together and came up with the following:-

1 He was from Egypt.
2 He was more than one but united.
3 He had killed Mickey.
4 He had got his son working for him.
5 He had promised the eight he'd sort Pete and Joe Bob.
6 He had blamed them for Nicola.
7 He would now not leave.
8 He had big plans.

Pretty useless. Pete thought he recognized a way. Let him think Pete was a follower, then try his patience so much that he goes nuts, give him poison instead of respect. This would be undercover and very risky. Yet Pete's motivation might drag him through with success. It was complex, passive aggressiveness with extreme prejudice. The professor had an idea. He did not really understand Pete's.

"All out attack is the way. We need to rally the whole community, and take away the people he rules and let them attack too." But although this was obvious he knew it was like attacking thin air. There was the need for skilled mind engineers, people who know how to work and shape the mind violently. People like Nile, he thought ironically. It had also been the Professor's job too, he didn't know of many with the same class of ability as his in City 29. He supposed he could make it international and employ workers from other cities.

Pete told him he was not prepared to be some general, it did not have a certain outcome, they could lose fighting him this way, then he would be even more powerful, no he could not risk it. His own idea would be the only way, he'd wait until he moved out, he would discuss it with Joe Bob.

"Shit." He'd asked him to move in, he could not go back on that. Oh well, he trusted things would work anyway.

It was dark out in the countryside. The Professor reversed and turned the car around and drove Pete home.

"Leave it to me, I'll help your son." Pete walked through the door past the office where Louise had just come on.

"Where were you?"

"Out for a walk." He carried on up the stairs and everyone was in the smoking room, for the tenants the hub of the hostel. They were nattering away, far away from the important business Pete had just left. He was happy to be there. He relaxed, he'd talk to Wolfie and Joe Bob later. He joined in the banter.

Pete sent out a vibe to Joe Bob showing him the room empty. They waited, Louise gave them their medication and they returned to the smoking room. The others did not bother them and went to bed. Pete smiled and as he rolled one he relayed his plan.

"Undercover, it's the only way. Of course you can move in but I'd like you on board, otherwise it could get complicated, what do ya say?"

"I don't know." He thought he wanted to move in with Pete but entering into a fight for other people's rights, he wasn't sure. He did not like to get in involved in society, he always felt it was watching him, Pete was different, he did not watch him and he suspected they watched Pete too. They'd still be friends after it. So the answer was "No."

"I just don't want to get involved. I'll wait until it's all over if you don't mind, then I'll move in, Padraic said I could stay here a while longer." Pete stood up and put his hand on Joe Bob's shoulder and said,

"Okay, no problem, you are a friend and we will party once

again and that's a promise." They went to bed and slept quietly and soundly.

The next day Pete went to the office and signed the forms that Padraic had filled in for him.

"Most of our tenants like to keep living in the south district, the west is a bit wild but you know what you want, we should have you moved out in a few days." Padraic didn't mind Pete, he did his chores and got on well with the other tenants, he was not a dope fiend like some of the people who passed through.

"So we will be on hand if you have any problems and please call round for a tea any time you wish."

"Cool, thanks a lot." Pete had other business today, lastly he had to phone Jackie and illustrate his plan of action.

"Hi, Jackie, Pete here, I need to meet, do you know..." He named a coffee shop in a trendy street in the city.

"Well okay, but I have to be back in a couple of hours, I am going out with Leo. He does not like me doing this stuff."

"Okay, see you in an hour then." He said goodbye to the guys in the smoking room and left. Joe Bob watched him from the window and sat down.

Jackie arrived first and sat on a couch. A waitress came over but she told her she was waiting for a friend. Pete came, he looked around and saw Jackie and sat opposite her. There were about ten different coffees and teas on the menu. Pete felt psyched so he took a pot of calming camomile tea while Jackie took a hammerhead coffee, that was an americano with a shot of espresso topped with filter coffee. Pete started the talk;

"Don't see you in the closed circle anymore. See you've taken the initiative."

"Yes there are four of us, we have been excluded from the circle, we want to create a happier society and that will mean fighting for your rights and making sure that that tyrannical eight does not return."

"Okay" said Pete; he felt that this fight of hers was against hypocrisy and to make sure the totalitarian state did not return.

"Your cause will be hard and full of strife, sometimes you'll be swamped and will feel like you have made the wrong decision" Pete prophesied. Jackie reflected and felt uncomfortable, she did not wish it to affect her home life as it would be impossible to lead a double life, one - loyal wife and two - defender of the people.

"Now," said Pete, "I called you here to let you know *my* plan of action. I am going to go undercover and join Nile."

"You are what?" She paused for a couple of seconds, "Why would you do such a thing?" Pete did nothing to counter her anger, he waited.

"It's the only way, I'll need your help, he may ask me to attack you so if you see me crazy, know that it's part of my plan. It won't happen until I move out of the hostel in a couple of days. Beware. And by all means keep doing what you're doing, your fight is a good fight." Pete then remembered that he ought to tell Alex and Kelsang. Kelsang would have advice for him, he was sure.

"One thing I'd say to you, Jackie, is to not allow your relationship to suffer for that is precious. Fight for it first, then fight for the cause." He sipped his tea and looked at his surroundings; he liked this place. Jackie was quiet as she was trying to understand what Pete had been talking about. He left Jackie with many questions and paid for their drinks and left for the east side to find Kelsang and Alex.

He decided to try Kelsang at his terraced house. The gate creaked and before he could rap on the door Alex opened it.

"Oh, hello Alex, glad I caught you, I thought I'd have to go to your house, is Kelsang here too?"

"He's at the community centre, he left me here. I've moved in with him to learn and be his disciple." Pete wasn't shocked. He said heartily,

"That's the business, Kelsang's a good person."

"Do you want some of his tea? He's told me I have to drink it every day." Pete had already had a tea but what the hell, he was on a roll.

"Okay, I'll have some." Alex turned and Pete followed him to a crammed kitchen. There were pot plants that Pete assumed were medicinal herbs. Alex opened a big clay pot and pulled out a bunch of reddish green herbs and put them in a pot to make an infusion. Soon it was bubbling away on the stove and that green steam started to erupt. They brought their teas into the lounge, incense sticks gave off wispy smoke and a peaceable smell that reminded one of strangely forgotten times.

Alex was sipping it with great relish, looking in the steam then looking up at his guest, smiling the odd time. They were sitting on cushions watching the smoke and drinking tea when Kelsang arrived.

"Ah Peter and my favourite disciple." He stood looking down at them and had a smile that was permanent as he knew how to keep all negativity away.

"So Pete has some news." Unfazed, he spoke.

"The demon Nile has taken out the authority and has taken a friend's son, as you probably know."

"Yes, I have seen this and you are going to act on it."

"Well I am going to follow him and bring him down."

"Okay, and you want my advice." Pete did not need to utter, Kelsang saw his reply and put his hands together and emptied his own mind.

"An honest motivation can hide the deepest of lies."

"You mean Nile won't know."

"In a way yes, if you keep straight." Alex sat watching them with wonder.

"So I can count upon your help?"

"You may. I don't know what will occur but you can rely on me."

"Thanks, you have put me at ease." And he stood and left. Their minds didn't follow him. He was on his own but was happy enough as he got on the bus back to the hostel. He gazed out of the window and watched the passing streets and run down shops of the east district. He saw a group of chavs at a street corner, he changed buses in the city centre and got the south bus. Not so many people on this bus. He got back to the hostel, it was tea time.

Four days later, days of keeping his mind calm before his great attack, Pete put all his stuff in a taxi and was driven to his new place in the west. The house was an old one, built for factory workers in the industrial revolution, many people had lived in it over the years. He had two bin bags of possessions, one with clothes the other with a radio and other essentials, which he carried in both hands. He jammed the door open with his foot and dumped the bags in the front room and paid the guy in the taxi. He was by himself for the first time in years but he had business to do. He got the radio out and sat down on an old discoloured armchair, the only thing left in the room by the previous tenant.

He drummed his fingers on the seat arm and thought.

"Well this is the time; it's now." He continued his thought, "Time to contact Nile." It was an easy act. Half a second after he thought of Nile he came.

"What the fuck do you want?" he cursed. Last time Pete

had beaten Nile and both knew that and also that Nile had framed Pete. But Pete had an approach he thought might work, he remembered Kelsang,

"Hey man I really admire what you do, the eight gave me real trouble, I want to rule, I know I could do better, I want the power and respect, I want to go with you." Nile searched Pete's mind but Pete had broken off all ties and this empty house was all he had. Nile looked, he was more happy than confused, Pete was a mighty sage and he'd definitely have use for him. Pete was his second follower, there was Voodoo man as well. He wondered how he'd take to having another person working with him, probably not well but he didn't care.

"Okay, you can come on my side but I demand devotion." He then left, he swished away, he was about eighty percent sure of Pete but that didn't matter, he being demonic felt invincible, he was that kind of a maniac. Pete was on his own, he still had to stay in character because Nile would detect traces of whatever he did by looking at him or the energies Pete left behind.

So he sat on his own for half an hour. Not much light shone through the net curtains. Also it was a depraved area, there were harmful entities in this community that fed off the poverty, drug users and the other social problems that existed there. He got off the seat, now his, and opened the front door and stood out in the street, a long street of identical terraced abodes. He closed the door and was outside, it was brighter but still dull. He went for a walk, not out of curiosity of the area but just to make things seem normal. Then Wolfie came, he told him to shove off and to stay in his own world for now, he hadn't thought it would matter to have him about but now he saw it could be dangerous. Anyway it would be a good effect for Nile to see the trail of hurt that Wolfie left, Wolfie would find out from the other side what was going on. He wondered how long this would all take, but he did not care though it would be nice to get back with Joe Bob. The world would always be a stranger to him, it no longer made him feel sore.

It had been an hour since Nile left and he took Pete unawares as he walked down a street two over from his.

"So how do you like your new area?" he rasped. Nile had often frequented this district, he had a network of like minded demons here, it could be a right laugh.

Nile crowded Pete, he wanted results and to make Pete see his vision. Pete knew his vision was crud but they strode back to his house, Pete with a smile on his face. He picked the key out of his pocket and sat down.

"I've just come from my other ward, I showed him who was now in the gang and he was surprised. He saw you with that other pal and can't believe you. You're up to something," he paused and looked at Pete and continued, "he thinks. But we'll soon find out whose side you're on." He left Pete. Pete sat down and thought a television would be nice, but he did not have time as Nile was back.

"Okay, get up. I need you to go to the north side. Your new friend is outside." Unsteady, Pete got up and gingerly approached the door. He could already see the outline of Voodoo man through the glass. Pete thought, "That cunt" but he corrected himself, he would not give himself away, this was his new friend. He flung the door open and heartily shook the other's hand. He was wary of Pete and did not say anything, he stood gazing into Pete's eyes hoping he would give himself away. He did not, so Voodoo man clutched Pete's hand and pulled him out of the door and they set off at a fast pace. He said,

"Listen we are going to the house of Nicola, one of the secret ruling organization. She's gone back on her word with Nile and he wants us to make our presence known to her. When Nile gets things going it will be good." Pete was unaware he'd stopped talking and Voodoo man was waiting for a reply. He psychically shouted out to Nile that this guy was no good. Nile was far off and had a look.

"He's just starting, give the boy a chance" is what he said.

They kept walking and got on a bus. Pete wondered if he'd ever be friendly to him. Pete made a move, not to help the sabotage of Nile but to fit in, to try and get him talking.

"Do you like the area? I think its got a certain community feeling about it." Immediately he detected that Pete was trying to lead him into conversation. Normally he would have scorned someone doing that with him, it was so weak, but then they were apparently brothers in arms now so he spoke. His voice was hoarse from days of not using his vocal cords.

"It's okay, I moved there to get away from the ruling psychic institutions and because people keep to themselves in the west." He thought about what he said to develop it but he suddenly saw he was being weak; as if he cared people kept themselves to themselves. Quite disgusted, he was quiet again. Pete saw, and said,

"Yeah, everyone needs a place to keep away from the sides." He thought this was down Voodoo man's street. He continued. "Yeah, a place that you can retreat to and that can't be penetrated by anyone." This rubbed him up the right way. He gave Pete a vibe of comfort and they sat back, slouched on the bus's seat. They began to talk just like they had at their first meeting in the Stevens ward. Pete liked the guy. Although he was going the wrong way in life he was civil and his intellect was engaging when it was shown. Perhaps Nile liked these parts of him too. The bus arrived at the changing point in the city centre and they got off.

They stood on the city square waiting for the north express bus. People from all over the city walked past them, not aware of them. The two watched these people, people in their own world with own their plans and it was apparent that they did not include Pete and Voodoo man, they'd been thinking together and laughed. Pete would enjoy his time here but he still had to beat Nile. The Holy Spirit would show him he trusted. Although Voodoo man was still reserved they kind of trusted each other, well as much as they could with all the business. The bus pulled over.

They sat together in the middle, both vegged out but Nile made an appearance and that put them on their toes. For the rest of the trip they looked ahead. Nile had shown Voodoo man where her house was, a mansion would have been a better description. It was quite a walk away from the stop, purposefully far, this was an exclusive area. A boy in a school uniform who was going home stared with suspicion at Voodoo man's facial piercing.

"It's over here, he told Pete." It had a high fence and the window was quite far but had its blinds up. Why were they here if Nicola could not even see them? But the other figure trusted Nile, it was dark now. They crouched down and sat against the wall but they didn't have to wait long. There was a scream and Pete and Voodoo man were mentally transported to the house. It was Nicola who had screamed, she was looking at her younger son who was pale and in his left hand he was gripping a knife that was dripping with blood and there was a dead animal at his feet.

"What have you done with the dog?" she looked at the boy; he was beginning to return from where he had been. It was Nile but he was not finished. He travelled and met Pete and showed him, Nile becoming a power in front of the eight.

"Do it" he said to Pete. "Use the boy." Nicola did not care

about the dog, she cared about the boy. This was too much, she'd only just recovered from an attack herself. The colour was beginning to return to his normally rosy face, then he barked and gave a grunted scream. Pete said,

"Leave the leadership to Nile, King of the ghosts, or we'll fuck with you." The boy fell down scared out of his wits, but Nicola surprised herself in that she kept control, after all she was ruthless. She knew who this Nile was, but king of the ghosts? Well their usual ones had left. And that voice, it was Pete's she was certain who it was, she pulled up the blinds and there he was, unmistakable. He stood at the bottom of the garden looking back at her. She pulled the blinds down again and went to her son. She would be submissive for now but they would be dealt with. Pete too was surprised at what he said, he liked the first part but was a bit shaken with the expletive he had used.

Nile zoomed over, he was pleased and said they should return to the west. They set off and strode quickly in the dark. Voodoo man was pleased the job had gone well though he was a bit jealous that Pete had done the job. He'd gone to jobs with Nile before and had never been allowed to intercede in such a way. It had been a long day. Pete's house was on the way to Voodoo man's and when they got there Pete said,

"Cheerio." and his new friend raised his hand up a little and walked off, into the night. Pete thought about the day, some crazy shit and he'd had his fair share. He went to his bedroom and sat on the bed and looked out of the window on to the street. It was around nine o'clock. A group of four or five youths walked past and stopped by his door for a sneaky pipe of an illicit substance. Yet they were quiet.

"It's that sort of area," Pete reflected. He thought about reporting to his contacts, he thought hard. But he'd come this far. The room was dead quiet and Pete didn't like this, he was used to company, from anywhere. He sat uncomfortable but purposefully still. Ten minutes passed, then twenty. No Wolfie, he had to work at this. He knew not to watch Nile, he did not take nicely to it when Voodoo man had. He was worried if he pottered downstairs he'd give something away. He had to watch. He began to feel clammy and got up. The only light on was one he'd left on in the kitchen so he felt his way down the stairs. He turned at the bottom and he was struck.

It was not Wolfie, it was a psychic attack, and it came from none other than Nicola and she was backed up by Saul. Pete swayed on his feet and struggled to a wooden chair in the kitchen upon which he fell down. Nicola faced him so close he had to tilt his head.

“What the fuck do you think you’re doing?” thinking her power still gave her respect. Pete did not care, he was a bit more wary about Saul who Pete saw had a better idea about power’s nature than Nicola. She was a career woman, she was on top, Saul was more, but Pete would deal with Nicola. How would Nile wish him to deal with them? This was important in Pete being able to beat Nile, he had to act credibly like he was fighting hard for Nile, then when he had Pete’s trust Pete would blast him, but this was far off. Keep his trust was what Pete thought.

“What the fuck do you want?” he said rudely. Saul watched intently, it was Nicola who took the lead. If she had really been there she would have strangled him, instead she snarled,

“You fucked with two members of my family.” Pete pondered if a dog was really a family member, it was Nile who’d done the dog anyway. He tried to sound obnoxious as a servant of Nile’s would,

“So.” Then he thought he ought to blurt out some rhetoric. Best do it in an exaggerated hyperbolic way.

“You will never bring the great Nile down, he shall rule, you had your chance.” He lay back a bit more on the seat. She took him seriously and was angry.

“Listen young boy you will never overthrow us, I want you out of the picture, this threat I will carry out, I am warning you I have people, I know people, your master won’t protect you. I understand that we have hounded you in the past and that must be why you are attacking us. Quit now and we’ll try and come to an arrangement.” That would be nice, he might even have been able to do some good with the “arrangement”, but his cause was higher. He couldn’t tell them, he felt mild pain. He hid it and said,

“No joy, no doubt I’ll see you and your crew soon, good luck.” He laughed.

“Why, you little shit.” She offloaded a lot of dark frustration and tried to hold the power she used to have, she was not sure if it was there, she drifted away.

Saul looked down on him and on their own he fixed his eyes on Pete. Pete looked back and Saul left. An emissary of Nile’s had been watching and he left too.

"Hmmm, a nice mug of chai." He got up and dug some out of a near empty cupboard.

"Shit, no milk."

Chapter 32
Movement Occurs

Three groups of people wondered how Pete was getting on; there was Kelsang, Jackie and her crew and the Professor. Pete cared about the Professor, he was a man who cared for his son and had made a stand against the authorities. Kelsang no doubt was keeping track of things and then there was Jackie's crew. They were the ones in most danger, being an active unit in this project. Joe Bob had watched Pete in the old manky house but had ignored the happenings and was now talking to Dwight in the Golden Horse, he'd just given in to a bit of harmless curiosity and was not really interested in how Pete was getting on, a far way off.

But the closed circle was not ignorant of Pete's activity. Eugene opened up the meeting. He'd called it.

"Well our group has lost members but that does not matter, we are still the official dealers with the other side in city 29. I have had Jeremiah watching them and he's sure they are up to something and we can only assume they are trying to take power. The ghost Nile is on the rampage and I wish to tell you the renegade Pete is under him now." This shocked them, there were eight of them left not counting the guides that each of them had. A thin grey haired woman wearing a woollen green jumper stood up.

"Yes Iris?" She had been in the circle for many years and saw their work as being of the utmost importance to society.

"The eight seem to be putting up a fight, should we be helping them?"

"Well no, I think we should concentrate on seizing power from the demon and when we have it we will return it to them, with our complements, eh?" Eugene already had information from his guide and he decided to share it.

"The ghost Nile has little support in his world although Nile seems to be at least a hundred strong, they are all warped together" (this scared him) "you see. Like Legion in the New Testament. Unfortunately we are not Christ so it will be hard then." He gave the impression of humbleness, that was far from true. But they were still recovering from the word that Pete had changed his allegiance.

"Joe Bob though has left Pete. They've parted ways, we can assume they have fallen out." It was Oliver that said this. Most of the others thought this was a shame as two friends had fallen out but Oliver continued,

"So Pete won't have as much power and that is good. We will leave Joe Bob to a later date. Heathcliffe has other info - Nile has another disciple, we are not sure of any name, he is a dangerous individual and you would think we would have had had dealings with him before but Healthcliffe says this one is extremely cunning."

Eugene then told them about the attacks on Nicola, how she recovered from the first one only to have her son attacked, it was all over the ghost world what had happened and the second one had included Pete. The rest of the circle were troubled that the situation was becoming more and more grave and with increasingly perilous consequences. Iris wished they were back to normal circle duty like helping spirit people in trouble, yet she trusted Eugene implicitly. He carried on with his report.

"Then there's Jackie and co, I have assigned a minor guide to watch them, at least her "friends" can no longer back her up." He meant Pete and Joe Bob of course. It made him and Oliver happy that Jackie's friends who had been the cause of her expulsion were now against them. Eugene tittered to himself at this.

Later that night Jackie told her husband she was going to play hearts (a fun game of cards a bit like whist) with her friends but she really went to one of her newly founded breakaway circle's houses. She was the last to arrive and was ushered into the front room where there were chairs arranged round a table with candles. They flickered as Jackie sat down. They all knew what not to say, the room had ears, as by a silent email they all knew the score, tonight was going to be an act of disinformation and a time to see how Pete was getting on, they might even make an appearance, yeah they'd run off with their tail between their legs, that would make Pete look good.

"Okay people, let's do the job" called Jackie. They began to think of Pete but someone did not want this - it was Jeremiah, he was trying to marshal their circle.

"Get back" he said in a quiet controlled way, but this only made Jackie annoyed, it was much like a parent telling a near grown up child to go to bed. But she knew the way to get past was act in a quiet controlled way. Some of the others were taken aback so she acted quickly, she sent out a vibe saying you have nobody else saying "get back" it's only you so "fuck off." Jeremiah concentrated on the others. He said out of Jackie's earshot,

"Leave this woman, go back to your lives. This business is being carried out by other people, there may be trouble but you have no need to get involved in this." Jackie went on to look at Pete but she didn't feel the full power of her circle, she brought her consciousness back to the room and one of the group stood up.

"I have to go" he said, and walked out. It was a guy called Andy who had joined around the time Jackie had. The others watched and sat stoically. Jackie stood up. She glanced around to make sure they were alone and said,

"We have to help Pete, nobody else is, yeah the others might be resisting the demon Nile but it is Pete who will destroy him, not Jeremiah and his pals." The three who sat around the table had had their enthusiasm renewed.

"So let's fight." Jackie said it like it was some politician's speech, perhaps it was. They did not need Andy. What should they do, the eight? The closed circle? Nile? Jackie knew, attack Voodoo man and let Pete beat them away, at least that was the plan, to make Pete look good.

They meditated for ten minutes to calm their minds then Jackie ended the silence with the ringing of a tiny brass bell. She spoke.

"Let us dwell our concentration on this boy." Their guides had a couple of seconds before zooming into Voodoo man's space. They followed.

He neither cried out nor showed aggression; they flew round his head like a swarm, then he looked at them. With hate he imagined them in as much pain as he could muster. They dropped like stones and landed in the bottom of Voodoo man's vision, but he did not call out to Nile, but went to stamp down on them. He was enjoying this anger. Pete though watched from afar but did not intervene, he was curious. Jackie watched the stamping and anger, she cried out the hate had isolated him he'd wanted it all for himself, so now he was alone. They rose quietly like flames and formed a circle around him before he could call out.

They watched him and saw a pathetic character, but Voodoo man was struggling to maintain his image of power, it was running off him like water. Pete jumped in and flexed his hands and threw lightening off them. It was only in the mind, the effect was an arrangement with them, Jackie feigned pain and they cried out and left with their tails between their legs. Voodoo man watched the power lightening represented and he respected such violence. Pete thought this might work.

They emerged in the lounge and Jackie said,

"Good job, I think that's it for today." They all went home as reward settled on their minds. Jackie got in and made coffee and sat down with her hubby to watch "Eastenders."

Meanwhile the Professor had been called to Saul's house in the north. He pulled into an apartment block's car park. It was well lit and he had been there before, years ago, for that Christmas drinks party. It had been good, Saul had got one of the best interior designers of the whole of city 29 to do his house he remembered, the party had been a right swanky do. He passed through the lobby, and got the lift up to the penthouse. Saul came to the door and he brought him in and sat him down on an Italian leather settee.

"Listen man, what do you know about Pete? He's attacked Nicola's family, I know it was him that changed your, ah, working habits, what do you know?"

"All I can say is that none of this would have happened if you hadn't sought Nile, it's Nile that's messing with you and it's him, if you want change, that you'll have to take on."

"But what do you know about Pete?" The Professor thought back to the talk he'd had with Pete. He knew the truth but Pete had told him to tell people that he had joined Nile to rule for power although it would be him to finish Nile off. Of course if he told Saul this it would jeopardise Pete, it would leak out, he was sure of that and then the work Pete was doing would be ruined. He felt Pete had more of a chance to get Nile than the eight did and if he'd attacked Nicola it was to this end.

"I dunno about Pete, looks to me that he's joined Nile." He waited, thinking Saul would ask about his son's involvement but he didn't seem to know.

"What about the Priest? I think he could be your only help."

"Well, I am friends with him. Originally he did a good job when he attacked Pete but as always Pete fixed it right up."

"Well you're asking my help now yet when I left you weren't so amicable."

"You've helped Nicola, you are no longer banished from the organisation"

"But there is not really any organisation left" he quipped,

but he was still angry; what a mess these people had made. Then Saul changed the subject.

"I called you here today not just to talk about this Pete attack thing but I need your counsel and help, I want to contact the Priest and his friend the businessman and I think it would go better if you helped me." The Professor thought, then said,

"Yeah, certainly I'll help." This would be fun, for the ghosts the organisation used to employ were good people, it had been a pleasure to deal with them previously and if they had heard about Pete's secret plan he knew they would not 'spill the beans.'

Saul thought in normal times he'd be relaxing with a spliff and listening to some classical music, but since his job's fall he'd been working and searching for answers. Should he desert the organisation and start anew? He would give the organization a good try first before that happened.

The Professor sat back in his seat and raised his hands and relaxed, searching.

"I will call him then" the Professor murmured.

"No need for that." Saul produced a black box like the in the conference room and set it on top of some magazines that were on the table. It hissed.

"I am looking for the priest." The other end spoke,

"He's on holiday." There was laughter.

"It's Saul here." No answer, just silence. The Professor stood up and introduced himself to the box.

"Ah, Professor, I know of you." He thought it was probably Wolfie and Mocto that had told people. But the ghost did not reveal these links.

"We know you're righteous and that goes far here; what can we do for you?" This was really rubbing Saul's nose in the shit, but he did not react, if it accomplished his need then that was okay.

"Well can you sort out a wee chat with the Priest?" Saul asked.

"Professor, you want to speak to the Priest?"

"If you could friend, please."

"I'll have a look for him." He was gone for a few minutes so to make himself appear hard and unaffected by this affront Saul began to talk nervously.

"Don't have any family, but I see plenty of fine women." He mentioned a very attractive newsreader he knew, status was second nature in Saul's life but having such a phone call away did not make up for this mess.

"I don't have a wife, I am a widower, though I have a son." Saul only listened to this out of politeness, if he had have listened he might have made the connection with Voodoo man yet he did not. He thought he should have known the Professor was widowed; you could tell he was the sort who did not want to experience the sort of pain of a broken relationship again. There was an interruption; the Priest had arrived.

"Ah hello Professor, I've been relaxing in the spirit world sun."

"Hello Priest." It was Saul, "Welcome to my house again." The Priest could not be annoyed with this, he'd been enjoying his time off from government work and was only engaging with casual acquaintances. The Professor was one of these.

"Okay Saul, I like you above the others in your organisation. But it's fallen apart and you lot are in sinking sand, aren't you?" Saul had to put his cards on the table now before this guy ripped further into him. He was very uncomfortable. So he thought here it goes, he thought he knew how to talk to powerful people.

"Here on the mortal plain we the people that govern and keep the city/world safe have lost control just by trying to keep delinquents in check. One of your delinquents has taken our legal rights away, he goes by the name of Nile, you know, I beg for some deliverance. He tried to help, as part of a deal. We were in a rush, now all our actions seem to run through him." The enormity of the situation was brought home; this had changed his access to power that he had taken for granted, he felt a lump in his throat, he had to return things back to normal.

"And you're with him Prof?"

"Well perhaps we could all come to some arrangement." The Professor said cryptically.

"Well I will have a think, seeing you ask." And the box was quiet.

"That's the best I can do for you, I must get on, it's late and my son needs me." So he left Saul with his box.

Chapter 33
Downfall of One

Alex was in danger but he'd never enjoyed life so much, he often stayed at Kelsang's house. His parents had met this Tibetan called Kelsang with a mistrust of foreigners but he was a kind man and they saw that he was protecting Alex from things, things the two of them had always been shielded from. Why was Alex not shielded too? He had been as a child. They were happy yet dubious of this new path and he often came home to visit, a lesser of two evils.

All was quiet in the east district at least outside it was. Inside many of the houses Kelsang felt swarms of domestic arguments and negativity. Kelsang encouraged Alex to send out compassion to the community, to help the people. Kelsang had compassion, he practised it and always aimed to increase it, to hoard the good karma it produced, it was a Tibetan joke that in a way this was a selfish act as the Buddhist did the good for his own good.

Kelsang had never told anyone, but in Tibet he'd had an experience in the late seventies of a run in with Chinese government, he'd been in a detention centre for ten nights but he was compassionate to them and mysteriously they laid off, they still badgered him the odd time, keeping an eye on him from thousands of miles away. Sometimes in deep sleep psychically they would reassert their power over him, power they had had over him in Tibet. He always woke up and shrugged it off, he would smile as he realised he was far away from this strange tyranny. Here in this city there were the same sort of operatives, only these people had less influence in open politics and daily life. It had taken Kelsang a while to adapt to this new way of life but certain elements of this country were still just as dangerous.

They hadn't forgotten to help Pete. Kelsang called Alex into the front room. It was dark outside but the little light there was gave off a soothing atmosphere. Kelsang had been meditating and was still sitting in a half lotus position on a red cushion. Alex sat down. Kelsang was quiet.

"What to do?" Alex said nervously, he knew he'd soon be part of something and was anxious. Kelsang saw this and said,

"Calm. Bad actions always decay, you can clean the decay out but that will decay too." He was lost in his thoughts. Alex was about to prod him, to see what he meant, but Kelsang was enlightened and impressive, he knew to stay quiet. Minutes passed, as Kelsang sank deeper in thought Alex thought he got more worked up. He came out of this and smiled, he had his hands together in a prayer position.

"Okay, I know what we'll do, I will send some of my personal friends over to pay a visit to this Nile, heh, heh," he chuckled.

"Do you need my help?" asked Alex. He'd like to help but if Kelsang didn't need him that was okay with him, he'd stay downstairs, but he was needed, the master rose and he followed Kelsang up to the top of the house, an attic room, it was kind of small, there was another ornate woven carpet made of dark coloured thread, and the statue of Buddha. Kelsang told Alex to get the place ready. Alex knew how, Kelsang had instructed him in preparing for such rituals. He lit several incense sticks and poked them into a holder then lit a thick church style candle. He took a bunch of sage which he lit and chanting a mantra waved its smoke. Finished, he sat down by the door and Kelsang came up in his orange monk robes, he did not acknowledge Alex. Alex had been told just to stay quiet and in the unlikely event Kelsang was harmed he was to help him and bring him back into the physical world by whatever way he could.

Kelsang began to chant a different mantra, one Alex did not know. They were sat in the correct positions. He chanted,

"Oom ah hom padma guru sedhhi hoom." The words took on a peculiar power. This was repeated for ten minutes then he stopped. Inside or perhaps outside his mind Kelsang stood in the Buddha realm. His soul was away in this place. Alex thought he'd never seen such strangeness and knew Kelsang was not in the room any more. Alex became lost in his own thoughts. From the ground around Kelsang four Buddhas rose, one in the north, one in the east, one in the south and one in the west. They all had donned the appearance of their earthly incarnations. Standing in the middle of the four he watched their heads, then their shoulders rising, then he was gazing into north's eyes. He smiled at his spiritual colleagues before he was taken away. He was with them in the sky heading for Nile.

They flew and Nile was outside a disused warehouse talking to a younger demon. This young one turned his back on the Buddhas and drifted away. Nile didn't want him to go, he called to him and the younger raised his hand but continued to leave. Nile controlled his fury and looked at these unwanted arrivals.

"You're looking at the new ruler of city 29; what do you want?" Nile had a fair idea that they wanted to chastise him in some strange way and that they had travelled far to see him, he wasn't fazed in the slightest, if he had have been he might have been able to run away and save himself from what was going to occur.

"We come here to see your mighty work" said West Buddha.

"I have one of them" thought Nile.

"We come to admire your way" said South Buddha.

"Well I should be admired" reasoned Nile.

"We hope your relationships will be fruitful" said North Buddha.

"Oh believe me they will" laughed Nile.

"And that you give people something they want for ever" said East Buddha.

"That's totally me." Nile thought of the younger demon.

And Kelsang said, "And I brought them here." Nile looked at them all and could not figure out who to hit first. The Buddhas watched him think this violence and aggression and they believed they had Nile now he'd expressed this hatred. It was casual for Nile to do this evil.

"You cry out" said East Buddha referring to Nile's wanton badness.

"No I don't." Nile refused, thinking himself in total control of the evil he spurned.

"You move into actions" said North.

"No I don't." He could not connect his singular hate to other actions, he was the hater, he was not some pawn. He did not have time to sneer.

"You watch yourself gather" said South.

"No." Nile spoke clearly this time, he did not want his own evil; he gave out bad, he did not take it.

"You only see that which concerns you" said West. Something was coming over Nile he could not see as for something to concern Nile it had to be worthwhile, Nile was barren in this respect, he was sinking, he felt a pang of terror. Then finally he heard Kelsang say,

"I laugh at you." Nile stretched his hand out towards him with a hatred he reserved for choice incidents but it did not work, he had talked himself into hell. How had this happened? He had foolishly shown them his naked spirit and was vulnerable. He was caught, his outstretched arm would only get so far then it would flick back like it was elastic. He looked at them and they seemed far away but as big as giants, he cried out to his friends, so loud the whole district should have woken up but nobody heard him. In desperation he thought of Voodoo man. The action was not some threat or demand it was a cry of distress, and it was heard. Voodoo man heard it. He had never envisaged Nile's destruction, he thought he must have been called to witness some ghost atrocity of some sort but he only saw Nile struggling, wanting help so he could retain his power. But Voodoo man was not quick to act. He saw the Buddhas with indifference and he saw Nile and smiled at him, Nile did not return the smile, he was alarmed, he was not used to this. Voodoo man had always had to struggle even in his badness and so Nile would have to struggle too, no one had helped Voodoo man out.

"Good bye Nile, if you ever return give me call." And with that Voodoo man never saw the infernal spirit Nile again. The Buddhas grabbed Nile and brought him to a lower realm, a hell reserved for such people. How would he ever escape it?

Chapter 34
Eye of the Storm

Pete sat in his house oblivious to what had happened. He sat up in bed and tried to match his gaze with any event's imprints in the ether, in the psychic world, in the hope that he might see or detect something, anything that would put an end to the uncertainty of his situation. He did not see so he tried to sleep, he woke up again and there was someone in the room, it was Kelsang smiling though he was only there for a second then he was gone. Pete was sure that something had now happened so he phoned Alex but there was no answer, then on second thoughts he corrected himself, he still needed to be careful as he was still seen as being under Nile's spectre. It might not all be over. He stayed up the rest of the night.

Later he sat downstairs in the kitchen at a table, he had a cup of tea in front of him but it was cold. He sent out a look at the Voodoo man, a psychic phone call and there he was. He seemed to Pete free; the respect he'd shown Nile had provoked bouts of paranoia in him about his future but now he did not care as much. Pete showed himself and he did not look to Nile, Nile was gone, he looked at Pete and raised his hand in a horned position and pissed himself laughing. It had been a long time. Now there was definitely something amiss. Pete's curiosity got the best of him; he searched for Nile and he could see where he'd last been at the old warehouse, but now there was only a plastic bag being blown in the wind. Deserted. Wolfie came from behind and put his hand on Pete's shoulder,

"Kelsang did it, that nasty mother is gone, do you believe it?" Pete was so happy he was back in the kitchen jumping up and down clapping his hands. Tomorrow would be a day of celebration, he'd call over to Alex and see how they'd done it then he'd call on the Professor with the news then he would pay an overdue social call to Joe Bob and the crew at the hostel. The early morning news was starting on the television, he'd get some sleep now.

But this nap did not transpire the way Pete desired. It was about eight o'clock. Voodoo man appeared. Pete still slept. A chat followed.

"Your friends seem to have done the job on Nile, I never did trust you but you did get rid of that woman who attacked me with the African, so I may have some use for you." The experience had had little effect on Voodoo man, he was still power hungry. Pete thought him a "maniac." Pete had not got rid of "that woman", it had been faked, it had been Jackie and her friends.

"Look man I have missed my friends, I was undercover and now I just want to take it easy. You do your own thing, I won't stop you, but if you screw with people like Nile you will acquire Nile's enemies. If you take it easy you can have my friendship. I am not going to start on anyone, good luck." And with that Pete woke with a start. He put Voodoo man to the side of today's agenda, he got out of bed and stretched, he still felt like celebrating so he walked to a supermarket and got some groceries and cooked himself a killer fry. He ate heartily. He phoned Alex and this time there was an answer.

"Hi Alex. Pete here." Alex told Pete what had transpired and Pete listened intently.

"Yeah great news, can I come over, are you at Kelsang's?" Alex said he was. Pete couldn't wait, he exclaimed,

"Okay I'll be over soon, say hi to Kelsang." Next Pete phoned the Professor, he answered the phone sleepily,

"Yes, who's speaking?"

"It's me, Pete."

"What are you phoning me for? This could be dangerous."

"Your son's out, Nile's gone." He dropped the news like a bombshell and the Professor was silent. Tears trickled down his face.

"There's a couple of minor points I need to tell you, I'll call later this afternoon." Before Pete hung up the Professor asked,

"Can I call round to my son?"

Pete said,

"I don't see why not." And that was that. The Professor could start again to salvage the relationship between him and his son.

Pete was feeling great so he ate into his food budget to pay for a taxi and thirty minutes later he was in the east district of the city at Kelsang's door. He was surprised when Kelsang himself opened it. He raised his hands in a prayer position. Peace first. Pete did the same.

"How about some of that tea, I've got a taste for it" said Pete, slapping Kelsang on the shoulder.

"Of course, Alex go boil the kettle and throw an extra spoonful to the tea pot." There was a shout from the kitchen,

"Okay, coming right up." Kelsang went into the front room before Pete and sat down on a cushion. As usual there were incense sticks smoking away. Kelsang seemed pensive so Pete did not speak. Pete sat on a cushion as well. A couple of minutes later Alex came in with a steaming pot of Kelsang's special herb tea. He put it on the hearth and poured three mugs. Pete admired its green steam and sipped.

"Plenty more there Pete in the pot." Kelsang called. Pete only thought about asking the two of them what happened last night, how did they beat Nile? But he did not speak. Kelsang was much more cleverer in all things and before he could articulate the words Kelsang had read Pete's mind and he knew that that was why Pete had called to the house anyway.

"Okay Pete, my four other Buddhas from my lineage in Tibet surrounded him and he drowned in his own bad karma." And that was it, that was the big explanation and Pete sensed he could not go into it any more so he sat drinking the tea feeling the holiness of the surrounding atmosphere. Pete lounged about as he sat on the cushion and tried to let this strange atmosphere seep into him.

"What about the disciple?" Alex had wanted to know all day so now Kelsang was talking about last night's happenings he felt it was time to ask.

"He was there but did not attempt to help Nile, he could still be trouble though if that happens it will be dealt with like Nile was dealt with."

Pete left after an hour, he detected that Kelsang and Alex had plans for the day. He couldn't afford two taxis today, he'd have to bus it into town then get another to the north for his other appointment. He thought about phoning the Professor and asking him to collect him but he decided to just get a bus, he did not want to talk of things of such importance in a car.

He waited a couple of minutes at a bus shelter. It was a hazy day, the sun could be seen through wispy clouds. There was graffiti and gang tags on the shelter. A bus came. An old woman sat at the front with a trolley and some kid who should have been in school was at the back. Pete sat in the middle and soon was in his own world.

Red brick houses flew by and a public park was driven past as they travelled into the inner suburbs, then the bus halted at the city square and Pete got off. The journey to the Professor's house was the same except the houses were nicer. Last time Pete had been here was to get to Nicola's house, he recollected that horrible incident in a neutral way. She lived three miles away in a different part of the North district.

Pete strode up a small driveway. There was a sand pit covered in old dead leaves and the house itself had flaked white paint that was partly hidden by ivy that grew up the walls. A nosy woman across the road watched him, suspicious of Pete who did not fit in in the exclusive north, but this was dispelled when she saw her neighbour welcoming him in. The inside looked like it would have been chic years ago, that was when the wife had been living, it had not been redecorated since. He offered Pete a coke and as they were in the kitchen Pete could not hold back.

"Nile's gone."

"You said that, I am so pleased, I am going to pay my son a visit just to surprise him, I will hug him and I'll never let go of him again."

"Er, that's the thing, he may not be mixed up with Nile but to put it mildly he still has a, an attitude."

"That's okay, I am just glad to have him back."

"All I mean is that in all likelihood he will probably be a bit cold towards you." The Professor stopped,

"But Nile's away."

"He stills sees the perils of the dark as tempting."

"I have to pay him a visit, I have to see for myself." The Professor got up and got his keys, Pete followed him the Professor locked up and they got in his car. He kindly dropped Pete off.

"Cheers." What would Pete do now? He wanted to enjoy himself once again, return to his renegade ways. Shit, he'd forgotten, he still had to tell Jackie. In his house he sat on the worn armchair and dialled her number.

"Oh hello Pete." Then she said earnestly, "Do you need any more help?"

"That's the thing…" and Pete told her all the news.

Chapter 35
Like a Phoenix from the Ashes

Back at the army installation there was a meeting being held. They were slowly reasserting their power as the psychic rulers. Saul was a bit dubious, he thought it could happen again but he did not mind being back. Nicola was not the same leader, she was more open in the chair. As usual the black box was on the table. They had come to the meeting to commiserate and draw up a defence policy. Nicola was thinking along the lines of forming some telepathic guerilla outfit. They had gathered round the table and a ghost who was usually banned from entering such conferences (for always messing about) with happiness for the fall and happiness for being part of the bigwigs' conference shouted,

"He's gone ye ha!" The spirit then wondered who he could tell that he had got past all the usual guards left. The eight could not believe it, they could not take it for the truth, was it real? Carson spoke to the box -

"Hello, anyone, confirm the news." The Priest had been relaxing. He'd been having a great symposium with people who held a similar philosophy to Giles Delucius on life for two days and he was still going, but he heard the cry from the eight. He talked on for another few minutes then sat up,

"I better go." He was a bit peeved. His friends carried on without him.

"Okay, okay it's the Priest here, what is it?" Carson tried to sound important but he fumbled. The Priest watched and listened with amusement. The bald man called Curtis exclaimed,

"Just cut the crap, tell us were Nile is and where we stand. Are we back in charge?"

"Dunno where Nile is, if he's not about, he's not about. Where you stand? Well you are gathered together in a room with some screwed up mandate you seem to have retained." Nicola tried to retain the decorum the group had lost since they had employed Nile.

Nicola asked, "But will you help us?"

"No, you screwed up the contract employing that devil so the answer is no." The Priest thought to himself that he'd probably return to the conference and secretly look in on them out of curiosity, after all he'd had this job for years, he would still do part of this job, he'd make sure that they did not engage with elements that could effect his world, but he did not tell them this though. As far as they knew they were by themselves.

"Please help us" cried Nicola in a way that was meant to make the Priest see her desperation but he saw through it, a sly lie. He shook his head and did not answer. The table was quiet although in a place they could not see the Priest watched, he'd leave his spirit friends for a while. Nicola was not fazed, she immediately pondered on the other thing she had in mind. She spoke;

"Okay, we don't have their help, let's take a break for ten while Saul and I talk about a few technicalities." There was a noise of shifting chairs on the beech panelled floor of the conference room and they filed out quietly leaving the new planning to Nicola and Saul, trusting quite naively that things would soon be back to normal.

Saul looked suspiciously at the black box but did not mention it. He said to Nicola,

"Okay, what to do?"

"I want Pete" Nicola stated. Saul knew she'd bring up this revenge before he had asked the question, he spoke in a way Nicola would identify with. He said,

"Shall we put the surveillance back on Pete?"

"Yes, at the very least." She was already getting back into the way of things. Saul indulged her new mood and continued,

"What about the other renegades, do they wait, is it back to business as normal?" Nicola thought about her son; although Pete had told her through her son that Nile was in charge she also believed Pete was to blame for making her dear son kill the family dog. Pete had been with Nile, the demon that had taken her power. Power was her religion. No, before things got back to normal she would fuck with Pete first.

"No, I want that boy to live the rest of his life in an institution when I finish with him." Saul blinked, she was looking at him intently, she was deadly serious.

The rest of the eight came back after the break and quietened down. Nicola started the meeting again,

"I think the most important thing today is to make sure that Nile does not return, to do that we have to attack Pete, he's the last pawn. He is the number one criminal in this state, forget the rest of them! Does anyone have any ideas on what way this should be approached?" Nicola could think of plenty of ways but she wanted it to be a governmental decision, one seemingly made by the group collectively so to distance herself from any failing in the revenge. The small bald man Curtis stood up and looked at Nicola nervously,

"Well first we ought to reinstate the presence we had before this terrible business." The rest mumbled approval, it was simple and not to drastic, they were wary of drastic actions, but Nicola was having none of it, she continued speaking as if everyone was on her side.

"Okay, good that's a start, we'll get Connor and that other guy on the job, they did well last time, and let's get someone into that hostel he lives in. I have had experience of tough nuts and if you get someone in their space it can be brutally effective, war games of the mind." She did not know Pete no longer lived in the hostel, there had been so much else going on. Saul told her.

"He moved out and lives in the west district now."

"Okay, then what else shall we do?" There was no reply. There was silence. Nicola was beginning to twig on to a plan of action. Saul watched, he noticed the strong perfume she wore and he could see a craziness in her eyes, a side of her she hid from everyone. She made a speech, it started calmly but she got more and more worked up

"We need to set up a new squad, one under us of course but one dedicated to attacking these types of minds. No more shall we seek the spirits' help, that has only proved we need to do the job ourselves, no more disasters, only clean efficiency and control. No longer will we be threatened by crazy heretics, by psychic bullies, by some acne troubled teens trying to make a name for themselves; this will happen no more in our city, city 29. My own child was attacked in a most brutal and despicable fashion, a mere child of eight." She began to sob. "Pete reduced our organization to tatters. If it happens again will we recover? We don't even know how Nile crashed. I need to appoint someone to help me with this, Saul?"

Saul looked around. What could he do? He decided not to contradict her, if he backed her up he was pretty sure the rest would follow, but he did not do it immediately because he did not want to look like he was under her. Some were also afraid of her plans but were scared to be seen as weak, but with all this talk nobody could think of any alternative so they held their tongues, for now. He folded his hands and twiddled his thumbs. He looked around the table. He was afraid they might face up to him and Nicola though if they did he was sure he could change sides and still be one of the main players, he was playing a serious game. Nicola began to think out aloud and began to rant.

Someone coughed. No one looked up, there was a lot of talking, they were bouncing ideas off each other, the person kept coughing, the talk continued as did that cough, he was brought out of his thoughts as he noticed the rest were quiet, that cough was coming from the black box. Nicola stared at it in disbelief, she was on a roll, but she gave way as she did not want to seem foolish if it proved important.

"Greetings circle." It was Jeremiah! The circle at the spiritualist church had sent him. They had also been planning, and their next step was to approach the other greatest power of the city.

"I come from an important group of sympathisers and we have been watching the sinister events of the last days unfold, dastardly as they were. There was Nile who has disappeared thank goodness but there is still the chance he will come back, is there not?" Nicola was interested but this was some ghost, a representative of a people who they had never been involved with so she snapped;

"And what are you to us?" There was silence.

"Well I've been watching you." Nicola turned red and shouted to no one in particular,

"What do we pay our people, what sort of ghosts do we have backing us up if some nobody eavesdrops on our meetings of great importance?" She omitted that the organization she chaired was still testing the water and reasserting its newly found power. A ghost, one who though neutral helped as a go-between to their two worlds, who had been shown to her the day she'd started many years ago, spoke;

"This is Jeremiah, he is important and powerful and represents the city's Spiritualist church." When he'd brought Jeremiah here he thought he was doing the right thing, but now he was worried. Nicola retorted slightly more amicably;

"Okay Jeremiah, we are in an important meeting trying to decide what to do…"

"With Pete, and other dangerous renegades?" asked Jeremiah.

"Yes." Nicola was beginning to get warm to Jeremiah though she still perceived this new possible pact as risky. She tried to stay welcoming, saying;

"We are in the process of getting a crack squad together,

and this one will be exclusively living, our contract with the spirits is at an end."

"Ah, but we are only guides and direct servants of our mortal friends. At the church it's them and not us guides who you would deal with. We sympathise with the need for a new crack squad, we could devote some time from our normal rescue meetings to an attack, we will even report to you. I could sit in on your meeting, I could even send my friend, the church president Eugene. We have influence in the community, we are the main go between my world and yours, when any business is instigated it comes through us." The possible power Jeremiah saw the circle could become was making him spiritually dizzy. Nicola intervened and said,

"Okay, maybe you will be of use, we eight have to discuss the matter and come back later and then we'll come to an arrangement." She liked the respect he paid to her. Jeremiah left. Carson saw this possible development as a great opportunity.

"Yeah, we will keep this secret, it will massively increase the scope of our intelligence staff. We'll blend our organisations together and soon we'll have a sphere of influence that should infiltrate all society." Now any doubts about the attacking of Pete had gone, the eight now all felt they were heralding a new epoch.

"And put Bazza and Connor on him, make sure Pete feels their presence." said Carson.

Chapter 36
Blossoming Friends

Pete was on the way to see Joe Bob, but although the bus journey took the best part of an hour he was so happy, it did not bother him. He was soon outside the door. Padraic was surprised to see him, he thought it strange that he'd nearly completely forgotten about Pete. He stuttered, then pulled himself together; it was only Pete.

"Come on in, they're upstairs, how's the new house?" Padraic asked.

"It's great, the area isn't the best but I've never had any bother at all. I am away to see Joe Bob and that" said Pete and he left Padraic standing at the door. He entered the smoking room and smiled, he'd forgotten a lot about the old place.

"Ah ha my main man, how's it going?" He gave them a hi five. Joe Bob was smoking, Dwight turned around and said "hello" with a grin.

"Ah Pete." Joe Bob said warmly. Pete's news would wait. They all headed out to the Golden Horse. Joe Bob could tell he'd accomplished the quest he had not got involved in, he was indifferent but glad Pete was back as Pete made his routine more interesting. Padraic had been trying his best to condition the adventurous part of Joe Bob's mind to be more submissive by mundane conversation and psychology he'd learnt from occupational therapists. He had Dwight, Ryan and Rhona disconnect from him. Since Pete had left they'd been unresponsive to Joe Bob, he'd tried hard to engage them and it had driven him to cry secretly. The powers hoped he'd blame it on himself and change accordingly, but he did not blame himself, he knew the game, stay yourself, that's most important. But he was with Pete now and he was able to relax in the bar.

"So Pete, what's the new house like?" asked Dwight.

"Ah it's okay, it's in the west, it's a bit shady but I have a whole house to myself. I live near that guy, you remember him that guy who met us on the first night we all came here?"

"Oh yeah" replied Dwight cheerfully.

"Drinks?" said Ryan to them as he went passed the pool table to the bar. Soon they were all round the table with pints. Pete put on Kate Bush again. He liked that track. Ryan did not like it,

"Why are you putting on that shit?"

"I like it" said Pete. That bloody blue sierra was pulled in across the road, but Pete sipped on his pint, he was inside, away from them for now. Again Pete was aware of major events going on with the two merging powers, that was Jackie's old friends and that one who had her dog killed. He was used to the threats that that car symbolized, he was used to people spending time on him without him knowing, he could detect it, ghosts would watch these people plotting against Pete and when they approached Pete all the goings on flowed into his subconscious which he handled, he had to. Revelations can not be hidden. A bigger threat was being born. Pete said to the guys that this local beer was hard to beat. Ryan said he preferred the premium lagers. They drank more beer, by the end of the night Ryan was saying he did like the local beer.

"Let's go" said Joe Bob. Pete and Joe Bob walked back with the others but the way they spoke the others didn't hear;

"That demon, he's out of the picture, Kelsang beat him down." Joe Bob smiled, pleasure emitted from his head like a shock wave, the whole block felt it. Pete laughed. They walked to the door.

"Okay I'll call in the next day or so. You can come and stay sometime, see if we can repeat Dj Nutts at the union eh?"

"Yeah man." and they clasped hands, "I will leave this place myself soon."

Filled with an excitement the Professor was in his car at a red light, he scanned through the radio stations and could not decide which one he should listen to so he turned it off. He sped off at 40mph down a 30mph street and slowed as he entered the worse roads of his son's district. He got there to the terraced house and pushed the car door open and bounded up to the door. As he did he saw him through the window sitting on his couch, he had the radio on and was writing on a note pad. The Professor wrapped the door in a cheerful rhythm and waited.

After a minute he was beginning to be worried and was wondering whether to knock again. The boy knew he was there, how bold he was, their eyes had met at the window. Then the door opened slowly and made a creaking sound that made him think of a Hammer horror film, but the boy who was behind the door topped the whole thing off, he was pale and gaunt. For a moment they again looked into one another's eyes. At least there was no sign of

Nile. Voodoo man spoke with his own voice which gave the Professor peace of mind, previously he had let demons slur all the niceties out of his mouth, not talking himself. The voice brought back memories of happy times when Voodoo man's mother had been alive. They began to talk.

"So, are you still out of the game?"

"Yep, been worried about you though."

"Yeah I am starting again myself." Both were starting anew. "The last guy was an old demon, I am better than that."

"Yes you are." said the Professor, misunderstanding him (he was saying he'd do better at being a demon than Nile had).

"Can I come in?"

"Yeah, sure." The radio was still stuck on Goldie Oldie Rock fm and there was a musky smell, the top of his hi-fi was dusty with finger prints marked on it, but apart from that the room was relatively tidy. He didn't have many possessions, just the hi-fi, a television, a DVD player and a few CDs. If he had had lots of possessions the room would have been messy. The house had come furnished but the furniture was old and worn. A small table was scored and discoloured, there was a mug of tea with an old magazine as a coaster.

"Can I sit down?"

"Sure." The Professor sank into the seat and laid his arms on the arm rests and smiled.

"It's great to see you son." The son did not stare but he gave the bare minimum of eye contact to his father. He thought about his dad's constant work for officialdom. He'd had a lot of time on his own, especially when his mother died, you would have thought his father would have shown him a bit more love then but he didn't, he just worked, and now his father had come over all love. Yet since their last meeting he had become his own master so if he wanted, he told himself, he could make time for his dad, no one was there to stop him.

They were quiet. The Professor thought he detected some love toward him in this man sitting opposite, he decided to ask for a mug of tea.

"Can I have a tea?"

"OK." His son left for the kitchen at the back of the house's ground floor. The Professor kept his seat, he felt the grunge music playing was inappropriate but did not want to turn it off. He heard a kettle whistle.

"You still take milk and no sugar?"

"Yes, you remember."

"And a rich tea biscuit?"

"Okay, go on." And they sat down. The father said to his son,

"Listen, I would have said this to you last meeting but you were not yourself. I want you to join me and fight for good things, I believe you already know Pete, he's a personal friend, we won't do anything too taxing, just test the water the odd time."

There was silence, then the colour came to Voodoo man's face and he gave a long thin grin and he laughed,

"Ha ha ha ha ha ." He laughed for an uncomfortably long time.

"Well?" The laugh turned to a titter, then he replied;

"No Dad, I think I will stay the lone wolf. I have no ambitions, I am on no sides, good or bad. I am my own master. I am mustering myself, the most I can hope for is that maybe our paths will cross." His father thought to himself that that was rather cryptic but he'd been called "Dad" - that was an improvement. He smiled back at his son and was careful to show empathy as his son still needed room to heal, but he would be part of that process now. Yes his son was definitely a strange one, he always had been, he'd always put it down to adolescent angst. Yet now he was a grown man. This was what Pete had been trying to tell him earlier that day. He wondered if he should leave, but decided to stay and see if he could prise any further love from his son. He had an idea,

"So you should see those bozos at work, they bit off a bit more than they could chew, completely levelled; one was nearly turned into a vegetable and now, well shit I don't know what they're going to do." Voodoo man thought and smiled again. He spoke, but again it was in a worn out way, he hadn't talked much recently,

"Yeah I always hated them, those drinks parties you used to have up north, so bloody sophisticated, not! They thought power came with their job, all so righteous. I laugh at how they fell apart." He was a bit manic, was this boy of his. He gulped at his tea and crunched on the rich tea biscuit. The boy kept talking;

"Yeah if you don't fight you will be ruled by people like your old work colleagues or you will be one of them, damn pricks." The Professor wasn't sure whether to agree with him, in the past it would have been an affront to be talked to like that. Sure, he was glad to be in his son's company but there needed to be a bit of work.

He told his dad about his plans, his quest and his new lifestyle he was doing it for the sake of it as no one was stopping him, not any demons nor the pig attitude his dad used to have when he worked. His dad replied;

"My new life consists of associating with whom I choose, it's a rich life mine, a life of no responsibility, does not that sound good?" He'd tried to elaborate but he knew he was trying his boy's patience. He could see the boy was beginning to get aggravated so he stood up and patted him on his shoulder;

"Bye son." Voodoo man did not get up.

"Bye Dad." The Professor felt he had proved Pete wrong with Pete thinking his son was still a maniac. The meeting had not gone completely his way, he would have preferred his son to be in a safer atmosphere. He drove home. Maybe he'd move to this area so he could be near his son. That Pete was a godsend. He could never have achieved his son's new freedom without him, and without Pete he'd still be a slave to the government. He was a happy man.

Chapter 37
Have Some of my Magic Beans

Trouble was brewing in the closed circle of the spiritualist elders. The meeting had not started yet, they were waiting, a car pulled up outside and a door closed. Someone opened the front door. Eugene got up and left the side room they were in. When he returned he was with a black man who (the spirit guides noticed) took in everyone in the room in with an unnatural speed.

"This is Saul" said Eugene, bringing him in. Everyone smiled, as they knew this man brought power with him. They politely waited, remaining silent.

"Hello, my name's Saul, as you know I am here as the representative of the psychic council and we hope to help each other for the purpose of keeping safe and protecting our country and its infrastructure from people wanting to harm it." There were murmurs of agreement. He then sat down, he could have continued the introduction but he wanted them to feel they had an input and to really believe in this new partnership.

Everyone introduced themselves. There was Eugene, Oliver, their guides, the old woman in the woolly jumper who was called Iris and the rest who stood up, saying a quick "hi." It would only be a matter of time before they had the power of this new arrival. Saul looked at them all and made it look like he was remembering who they where. After all, they were now workers for a common cause. Of course Saul thought this was a load of rubbish but he began.

Oliver spoke in opening.

"Okay friends, where to start, shall we see what you can do with Pete?" Oliver spoke confidently.

"Actually no, we ought to start with some of his cohorts, people who actually used to be in our own circle and serve Pete" said one of the lesser members of the circle. Saul was taken aback, he had wanted to be in and out, to get a game plan established and leave; no such luck.

"Okay,go ahead then" he said. They had been expecting some official help, a new injection of power. Oliver had hoped for more from this heavyweight official.

"We rather hoped for your help and contribution."

"So you want to attack this person?" asked Saul.

"People" corrected Oliver.

"Okay, you need to assert badness on them then curse them" Saul said. The circle were not used to this, this dark magic, it was crude. A gentleman called Arthur sat at the back. He observed and guarded the circle activities but he took the lead, Oliver watched, Arthur was a protector, he always kept the circle on its business, a kind of bouncer. Although Oliver always took what he said seriously, quiet as he was. Arthur stood up and said in a stumbled curse;

"Right, I will explain what I do and you can help. *Jackie the isolation you seek to carry out your business will destroy you.*" He paused and raised his eyebrows in a strange way; nothing then.

"Oh, ah yes that's the way to do it." said Saul encouragingly. Arthur continued,

"*And may your husband not see your soul and forget the love you share.*" Saul thought this was extreme, these people did not realise the laws of karma, they would get in a lot of trouble and difficulties, they had to be exact. But what could he say? He was nothing to do with them, he was just setting them up and they could go screw themselves as far as he was concerned. A bunch of power hungry idiots, they would end up losing everything, everything they had established, with this new drive for power.

"Okay," Saul said, "That's the sort of thing, though Nicola wants you to get Pete with us" He stopped, he needed to reassert the nature of their new relationship before he left, they had to stop Pete, that was all he wanted, maybe if they proved successful he would treat them seriously.

"Look I am only really here just to introduce myself and my associates in a face to face way, we meet every morning at eleven o'clock and each evening at seven o'clock excluding Saturdays, unless it's an emergency. We have certain dark technology that means you can talk to us through your guides, at those times. If we need you outside these times I will phone." He then produced a black box out of a bag he had brought.

"This is for you…" he explained to the circle how it worked.

Chapter 38
Looking Around They See...

Wolfie was worried. He had been snooping around the area of the spirit world the Priest frequented and was surprised not to be confronted by any go-between government cronies. It was like they'd never been there. Wolfie watched as various ghosts soared through to meet different vibes and quests. Eventually he tracked down the Priest who was watching a kung fu film on some sort of spirit television.

"Yeah man what's happening? How's the business? Looks like you'd never been there at that conference room." The Priest was peeved, he loved kung fu films and he'd had to pull a lot of strings with the Asian ghosts to get it.

"Yeah" he grunted, and went back to watching the film. The bad guy had just back flipped and kicked the hero at the same time. Cool. Wolfie knew he was annoying him so he hung back and watched the film. He watched it until it was over. He was sad it was over, where had he been all his life? These films rocked, but he had business. Finally the Priest spoke,

"Yeah, I still look in on the eight from time to time, seems they're going it themselves with some low rate spiritualist outfit, the leader's very pissed off with your friend, they've declared war on him." The Priest watched the blank television and stood up trying to will another film unsuccessfully. He muttered a goodbye and left Wolfie by himself.

"Shit, it is not good that they are concentrating their efforts on his friend Pete." He had to tell Pete. Pete was sitting on his ass watching an American comedian, he was cracking up, he was laughing so much the guy next door had started banging the wall,

"Shut up you spoon! Or I'll be round and make you." Pete shut up. He got up and pulled across the cheap net curtains that came with the house. The programme was over, the credits were rolling. What to do now?

"Pete, Pete have I got some news to tell you, you wouldn't guess what they are doing. You have to phone them." He looked.

"Oh hi Wolfie, what's going down?"

"You've got to phone the eight, they blame you, they think you're going to resurrect Nile or something. Here, phone them now, I have the number." Wolfie earnestly prodded Pete.

"No." said Pete, "I am not going to do anything of the sort, if they fight me they fight, they won't win." Wolfie could not believe what he was hearing, he had thought it would be simple.

"Well, if you don't I will." He told himself he had to approach these spiritualists, the eight would be guarded more but he'd try that too.

He went to the circle. Usually if you wanted to do business with them it was easy enough, that's what they were there for, to help relations between the worlds. When he got to the queue there were several ghosts there, more than normal, all crowded around a black box like the one the eight had. One said to him,

"There's a bloody queue here with this new box thing, I don't know what is going on, I have been waiting for hours, most of the people have left but I need to talk to these guys and their new box…" Wolfie left; this was proving difficult. Okay, he'd try the other black box. He got to it but since the word went out that the official ghosts had terminated the Covenant there were people playing jokes on the eight or asking for favours.

"What's the first thing you say when you get out of hell?" There was silence on the other end,

"Hell - low, get it." [Hello]

The eight got sick of these jokers and they turned the box off. Just before they did Wolfie could hear Carson say,

"Turn that thing off." Nicola said,

"We have to get the circle to send some heavies over." Then silence. He projected his consciousness on the meeting. He could see the room, they were talking about security precautions, they were thinking of Pete's demise. Leaving, he thought he might as well call on Mocto. This was easier as Mocto was pleased to see him.

"Hey Mocto man."

"Hello." Mocto looked happy, but he had not been doing much.

"Yeah since Kelsang came he (Alex) spends a lot of time in mindlessness meditation. I still love him but I'll probably move on, find someone else to help."

"Well you should see what I've got to deal with…" and he told him about the mounting attack that was about to be done on Pete.

"Well shit man, I'll help you out" Mocto said immediately. They met at a place were they could discuss things.

While Saul had been telling the circle about psychic attack, Jackie felt like someone had just walked over her grave, she was in the kitchen of her house marinating some fish with a peri peri mix when she felt her knees turn to jelly and she fell, it was a minor black out; she got back onto her feet. She felt dazed but kept doing her fish.

She felt someone put their arms around her waist,

"Hi honey." He kissed her neck.

"Oh hi Leo, love, I've cooked your favourite, peri peri fish and spicy couscous."

"Yes, I love that." They both remembered their honeymoon in Jamaica, and they were still in love. They both needed each other, yes the new circle engaged a lot of her time and its fight was important but she couldn't bear the feeling of being apart from him, or beat the feeling of lying next to him, and the love making. He was not aware of the responsibility and danger she had let herself in for, he thought she was just hanging out with that bunch of cookie superstitious friends looking at tarot cards or something.

They ate their meal and were drinking some red wine and frequently gazing into each other's eyes. Then she felt she couldn't link into the pleasant atmosphere, she could not grasp her husband; although she could see him, he was apart. Leo was savouring the fish, he was pleased she had cooked it but in her head she could not bring herself to ask him. Suddenly she heard from nowhere

"You are the first to go."

"The first to be neutralised by the new government." Again from nowhere. She was deeply disturbed. Where was this coming from? She recognised the voice, it was Heathcliffe backed up by Oliver. She knew and saw them sitting round that table in the back room in south district. The fact that they were messing with her with their hateful intentions made her panic but she could not betray this panic to Leo. She ate her food with a wry smile on her face. Leo was talking about a friend who always cracked him up, his mate Browner, he was telling her how he was heading out tonight with him, he laughed. With effort Jackie said

"Yes, and don't be back late." She put this in to keep a current of normality for herself. They finished their meal and the spirits were still messing with her, they were threatening any future spouse of hers now. She felt a cold sweat. Leo picked up her plate, she'd left a bit of fish.

"If you don't want it I'll eat it." He forked it into his mouth. He was in the kitchen now washing up, he had the television on listening to the sports news. She could hear the clinking of crockery. She sat slouched back in the chair,

"Just you wait…" went the cruel voice Leo could not hear, "We are only started." She left the table and went upstairs. She walked to the window, the street she saw could not hear what was happening. She gazed. Leo shouted a goodbye and she watched him walking away, down the street. She felt sick and picked up her phone and dialled the number of her circle. She knew her friend Mary would be supportive; the other two would back her up. It would be a simple school yard fight and these fanatics were not going to win. She told each of her own circle on the telephone of the attack that she was suffering at that minute and they were on their way. She sat down on an antique chair she had inherited that she rarely sat in and saw the attackers acknowledging her friends were on the way. She saw they went for the youngest of her group, a Chinese guy who was driving a few streets away, they showed him the attack on Jackie and laughed at him and moved on to him like Nile had done to the nurse Mickey now a few months ago, they now called Jackie's friend weak and useless. He doubted this was really going on but he could not find a welcome place in his mind where he could escape to. Then luckily he was at her door, she brought him in, he was shaken and as he came and saw Jackie also hurt a tear came to his eye.

"Come on in Julius" Jackie welcomed.

Mary arrived. She was one of the mature members of the original group, the one who the original circle had valued the most out of Jackie's group. But Heathcliffe and the other guides now looked at Mary with contempt, there were lots of her sort in their world, powerful types they could usually manage. They no longer liked her. They had tried to disgrace her and make her seem like an idiot to any of her dead associates. She'd already been fighting quietly for a couple of days. She was now aware that battle had commenced, things were changing, but she did not know about Saul's meeting.

She brought in an aura of calm with her. As she entered the room Jackie forgot everything and smiled, then she was ready.

"What the fuck do you think you are doing?" she said, looking at the marauders. She motioned to the rest of them and they looked at Jackie's attackers in a detached way. In their collective minds they stood together hand in hand and Heathcliffe tried to stare them down, but they were together and they were not going to be put down by their old friends.

Chapter 39
Trying to Get One's Head Together

Pete would loved to have helped but as often he did not know what was happening.

"Me part of Nile?" He thought back to Wolfie's news.

"Well I might as well have a look at things." He glared at Nicola's eight. Wolfie was right, he could see Nicola was infuriated with him, he could detect that she had been in deep thought about him. He tried smiling at her but her hate was too thick. Maybe he should call round, Wolfie had suggested this but Pete had not seen the point. Now he saw he wished to save her from this hatred, he cared about her inevitable pain. He made a plan, he'd go and see his friend Joe Bob. Joe Bob might be a layabout or kind of withdrawn towards important affairs but he had peculiar powers with regards the mind's realm that Pete was in need of. He found this urge to meet him a comfort, he thought about Joe Bob and he pulled himself up and set off.

It was latish, he was outside, catching himself off guard he regretted that he'd moved to such a run down area and had to remind himself he'd moved here because it was away from the influence of his enemies. He strode down the street, he walked passed the blue sierra now in the west and tapped the window. Bazza glared at him, he'd heard about what Pete did to Nicola's boy. Connor did not look at Pete, he had always thought he was okay, an innocent caught up, somebody who had brushed up bureaucracy the wrong way. Some of the organization had shared Pete's view about not needing the monitoring nature of the state but not now. They'd all heard about him and any love for this rogue was gone. The talk was that Pete had wanted the power of Nile and disposed of Nile, it was only a matter of time until Pete began getting disciples, a new dangerous power that had to be stopped. Pete knew he was being blamed but he had no idea it had gone so far in influencing people to rise against him.

He walked the mile down the terraced streets to the bus stop. The blue sierra was hanging back, knowing Pete's habits they knew where he was going,

"They are on the ball tonight" Pete thought. He clambered on the bus and it rumbled down the street. There was Voodoo man coming out of a tobacconist's, Pete banged the window and Voodoo man gave a wave. That put a smile on Pete's face for the rest of the journey. He changed buses in the city and got the south bus. He arrived at the hostel and was let in. He went up the stairs and found Joe Bob. Pete said things were good. Joe Bob said,

"They are not Pete, they have said you are a warlock, a necromancer, a danger to society. I have seen it. Sit down for a bit, hang out with me." He looked at Pete, and shook his head.

"I was not present when you went on your quest to defeat Nile, I doubt therefore I will fix it." He was quiet again. Pete could not tell what was on Joe Bob's mind. They sat in the room in each other's presence. Pete wondered if Joe Bob could tell what he thought. Though he did not feel threatened, he knew there was something funny about Joe Bob, he never prised out what though. He was happy to be worthy of being a friend of Joe Bob's. People sometimes thought that of Pete too, it was a responsibility he reflected humbly.

As Pete sat there he began to feel paranoid, he suddenly realised the impending danger and he did not think a chat with Nicola would rectify the situation. She was caught up in hatred and she was now blind to its recklessness.

"Shit" he thought. He watched Joe Bob and felt a cold sweat run trickle down his back.

"What to do?" mused Joe Bob. He drummed his fingers. Both he and Pete emptied their mind in desperation and sat in the room. Pete felt slightly detached from the situation, it was all quite surreal. He had to think. It was a problem like any other, he was engaged in solving it, he was no longer in the room, he gazed and saw Nicola a leader no longer needing the help from the Priest, she was a snake which could only be caught by a dangerously grabbing for its head, then there were the rest of the eight who buzzed about searching, searching for ways to hurt him.

The Professor was in his debt, but he had stopped his alliance with Nicola, he was happy but he did not want any more contact with the eight, he wanted to build on his relationship with his son. Thinking, he did not want the Professor to have any more contact with this dangerous snake anyway.

"What about Jackie?" Pete was shocked, Joe Bob had been reading his train of thought, before he could look Wolfie was beside him and told him that she was the one to seek. So seemingly it was only these friends on his side against the whole world. Joe Bob stopped him being frightened, for now. There was someone else in the room,

"Time for you to go Pete, it's medication time for Joe Bob." said Padraic. Pete went down the stairs. Louise was in the office, Pete poked his head in.

"Ah Pete how are you, you settled into your house? The nights have been all quiet without you." Laughing, she was happy to see him. Pete made her feel that she was worthwhile as Pete liked her too. So Pete told her about his new digs.

"…Yeah, it's in the west, not as posh as this hostel."

"Oh, I used to live in the west, though when I got married I moved to the north, better schools for the kids there."

"Oh well, cheerio." And Pete was off into the free night, at least that is how Pete would have preferred it. But outside waited Connor and Bazza, they followed Pete at his walking pace then they sped up and swerved in front of him. Pete stood and watched, ambushed. He was kind of bemused. These guys, what did they want? Bazza got out of the car and strode towards him. He pushed Pete with a shove, thumping his collar bone,

"We know you; we might not be able to fuck with you, you being so blooming clever, but you better make sure, you watch yourself, we are not going to kill you." That would not solve anything, he told himself. "You'd probably still screw with us, no Pete we are going to pulverise your mind." He thought his words awesome, he looked at Pete, he'd been following this boy for over months now and he thought him pathetic. Pete had put all his mind into being powerful. Most normal people just let things happen, they lived and breathed in their own circle of close friends, and were happy. He, Bazza had his own family, he hated having to bother with Pete, sometimes he felt he'd liked him but since he'd gone to Nile's side he was faithful to his supervisor's policy and would fight him tooth and nail.

He glared at Pete. As he'd been thinking he did not realise he'd squared up to Pete. Bazza had a chubby face which had gone a ruby red colour, he had no respect for this scrawny boy, the boy had gone out of his way, trying to bring down society. Bazza was getting worked up now, he had to stop this, he raised his fist and swung at Pete who dodged out of the way. Next thing Connor was beside him, he had an arm round him, he also looked at Pete with hatred. Connor spoke gently,

"This isn't the way Bazza, come back, come now, take it easy." Next thing Bazza had come round and was in the blue sierra car.

Pete walked to the car and tapped on the window. Connor wound down the window,

"Any chance of a lift?" Now Connor was annoyed and Pete was scared! He floored the car and was away, they drove round the south district and neither talked, gradually they relaxed and decided to get back to the job. They drove to Pete's street and waited outside. He didn't return home that night though, so Bazza and Connor sat waiting.

At the same time Pete did not want to go home so he walked to the east, to the monk's house. It was a long walk and as he walked in the south it was pretty deserted, just the odd taxi flew down the tree lined streets. They were also well lit. This changed as Pete entered the east district, this had taken over an hour and a half to walk. The east was not so nice and Pete was a bit cagey, he walked past a public house and a group of men stood outside smoking. Pete thought they would come over to him and ask him his business, but they just stood silently watching. Pete walked faster. He walked past a church, its old bricks were covered in green moss and the grounds where quite overgrown but there was a sign saying services were still on Sundays at eleven.

Then in another half hour he had made it to Kelsang's. He could see candlelight through the front window and he thought that Kelsang would have heard the gate creak. Anyhow he waited at the door and then after a minute he softly tapped the window. The door opened and there was Kelsang. It was around midnight, he did not speak but ushered him in. They sat down on cushions in the front room. The statue of Buddha had lit candles around it. Kelsang did not really seem to be looking at anything, he just sat with a slight smile. Then he spoke,

"Ah your friend is not here, he's home but I don't think you came to see him. Did you?" he referred to Alex.

"No, I seem to be in trouble, I did what I did for the good yet they don't see that and they hate me."

"Does this bother you?"

"No but it limits my movement. I have not lost any friends. I feel that the people attacking me could be spending their time doing things really worth while and this bothers me. I sit back, I like to watch the world yet it won't let me look, it stares right back" said Pete, trying to express the dire straits he was in. He felt cold.

"Oh dear. Well people often come to me with problems and I think I have a solution to yours." He paused, Pete looked at him, begging him to carry on.

"Give them a reason to come after you, ha ha, have a good time while you do it. Yes, ha ha ha." Pete did not see a funny side or really understand how to have this good time, but he would try. Staying here with the wise Kelsang he'd find the solution, he knew that, so he sat back on a cushion against the wall. He was happy in this room, the compassion of Buddha soothed his mind. He forgot about those guys, the ones that had squared up to him, he forgot about Nicola and her henchmen whom he knew wanted to hurt him, and he forgot about his bad times with Nile. He sat there in Kelsang's company all night, they did not speak much, they just sipped the special herbal tea and watched the flickering candles. Then dawn approached and there was a bit of light outside. Pete got up and he told Kelsang,

"I am off home, thanks I feel a lot better." Kelsang also got up and followed Pete to the door, Pete looked back as he opened the gate and Kelsang bowed. He'd filled Pete with new zeal. He splashed out and got a taxi home. The men at the public houses had all gone home hours ago, a man on his bike was cycling to an early shift at work. He slumped into the seat. The taxi driver said,

"You're out late mate." Pete just said he was, he was tired, they arrived, he tipped the driver a quid in case he thought his quietness rude. He opened the door, he thought a new door was needed, you could easily kick this one down. He got into bed and turned on a digital radio and as the morning news came on he was asleep.

Chapter 40
On the way home just a couple of things I have to do

Far away in outer space a lone spaceman of Mayan Indian origin was in a free planet trying to get his head around a virtual reality pinball game. This port had a game centre with many games from many worlds. The Mayan – Imoonan - still thought the Chinese game of "go" was the best, this was proved by the fact that it had been created independently in hundreds of worlds he'd visited, though the amount of squares on the board varied. He gave up on the pinball. The human mind did not have the reflexes of the few alien minds that were needed for the game of pinball.

He glanced over to another machine being played opposite. A couple of children were watching this guy, he could influence the trajectory of the ball. He was probably shit at "go" though, he thought jealously. The guy finally lost as the last ball went down the grate. He took off the helmet used in the game (the helmet detected the eyes' movement which in turn controlled the flippers that hit the ten balls that flew down different holes and obstacles). Imoonan shook his long hair and looked over at this pinball champion - his eyes had no irises, they were pure black. No matter how often Imoonan met people with different physical attributes it still disturbed him.

He turned and walked to the door with his back to the guy, even though he could not help being disgusted it was still seen as incredibly rude to be repulsed at diversities of appearance. He left and walked to a different building down a pebbled path. It was dark and he could see an outline of one of the world's two moons. He entered a cafe and sat down. He drummed his fingers on the counter, he spoke in a kind of Esperanto universal language that only was able to convey commands as different races could never understand the intricacies and views of others. Why so few could understand one another? It was just the way God had created the beings.

"One human coffee." said Imoonan.

"We have freeze dried, it's passed its sell by date."

"Okay." It was poured into a paper like cup. He went to a table and from his pocket took some powdered milk, the equivalent here was thick and its flavour had a bit of a twang. He also took out some artificial sweetener, here that cost the same as the coffee.

His ship was parked in the collective hangar a few miles away but he did not want to go back, he was lonely and had nothing better to do but to hang around here. He was waiting for someone anyway. The last family reunion he had been to had been long ago. His sister worked in the earth diplomatic service, it was pretty low key, her job was to exchange delicacies with other worlds and initiate trades and technologies agreements. She did not really have a boss of sorts and she got paid on amassing things she thought people on earth might find interesting, but she was not the only one doing this, so most of the time she brought back stuff the earth contacts already had. It was frustrating; she was hoping for the big one, if she brought something new she'd have the rights.

But the Mayan Imoonan at the cafeteria did not need to bother, though he did trade, he had a couple of kilos of garlic bulbs and chilli peppers that he was to move, that's why he was there, he had an alien contact who would exchange his garlic/chilli for some psychoactive leaves and cuttings that were obtained from a closed world that officially did not have any contact with others, this was difficult enough but the leaves were also illicit in that world. He would then return to earth and land at the travellers' airport in Nevada were he'd set a bribe in place so he could go straight through customs and meet another contact who was an agent for a pharmaceutical company.

Then in turn he'd be paid in American dollars which were good in many worlds. But he would have to spend about a quarter of the money on his ship's oxygen generator, that was an expensive repair and it irked him to spend so much of his earnings to fix it. Lost in this daydream he was tapped on the shoulder which gave him a jump.

"Shit." he said. The man smiled a mouth full of teeth and laughed.

"Shit." The man echoed in an odd murmur.

"Come back to hanger 13f and I'll sort you out, you have my stuff?"

"Yes, fresh yesterday." He showed him from a rucksack a shoe box sized metal box, it was cool to touch and it emitted a quiet buzz. The leaves would stay fresh in this "atmos box" for another week. The hangar was a couple of miles away, they walked, his contact sang a jolly ballad and laughed heartily. Imoonan did not know why he sang so. They reached Imoonan's ship and he exchanged the couple of boxes, he thanked the guy in the common language and the guy laughed.

"I like food," he said.

"Yes, goodbye" said Imoonan. He then picked up "The Outer Patriots of Earth" newspaper. It got some of its information from selling bugged black boxes to the authorities, also as earth life was growing outer patriots were often asked for advice so this was also leaked into the paper. Imoonan the Mayan spaceman thought his life would be a lot easier if Earth turned into an open world, and it was such possible developments that often made the front pages of the paper. Its journalists were quasi spies, the paper could not be touched by Earth's authorities, it was way out of its sphere of control.

The front page read "PETE SCREWS WITH GOVERNING INSTITUTION." He scanned the story. The Mayan chortled. That was the sort of news he liked, the whole front page was dedicated to this guy. He folded the paper and set off for Nevada. He loved the g force of a take off but the journey would be a long and tedious one.

Chapter 41
The Lower Powers Begin to Walk

At the conference room in city 29's military installation Nicola spoke. Jeremiah was in the box unaware he wasn't the only one listening -. a journalist in an outer patriot safe house was eagerly taking notes. Nicola was talking;

"...and if this works we will be the template for cities all over the United Kingdom, then perhaps the world. Bazza and Connor have been doing well. They've stepped it up a gear, we won't be toyed with." She surveyed the room; Carson was totally on board, Saul her number two was now being her whip but she believed that it was not really necessary, everyone was on board. The small bald man Curtis had made it clear to everyone that he was giving his total dedication and he would not stand for anything less from his other colleagues. He expressed this by showing complete glee as Nicola described the new template.

She talked about the spiritualist alliance and the words "here, here" came from the box, that was Jeremiah, they also had a living member of the spiritualists at the conference, Eugene was at the table, he had a big smile on his face, he liked the new partnership and saw it as a new movement of security, and he was pleased to let Nicola's organization control it. He liked the idea that he was just there in an advisory capacity.

"Okay, we might get Pete even with Bazza." There was laughter as they had read Bazza's report on his loss of temper with Pete the other night, he had been told the behaviour had been completely understandable.

"We must keep city 29 safe." Nicola paused for dramatic effect;

"I propose street wardens, to be made up of both church members and our own trusted people. These people will nip our psychic offenders on the butt and pass anything serious to district wardens who will link with other wardens before it reaches us - the higher echelon. A shared community. If I can prove this works then this will be global. We will confer with other cities and form world policies for the good. No longer will we be tormented by a bunch of nobodies." Moved, Carson banged his fist on the table. Eugene felt he was really witnessing something here.

"And as a reward for their dedication I propose we promote

Connor and Bazza to be the first district wardens. Their old posts in this new controlled society are no longer needed." she turned towards Connor and Bazza and continued,

"I know you won't let us down."

From afar the Priest observed, he looked at it all and said to no one in particular,

"This reminds me of Mao or Stalin." Of course the new council could not hear this and had they they would have seen him as a suppressive person out of synch with a new developing reality.

Over the next days the infrastructure was being born. Bazza approached friends in his area whom he deemed right for the job as his street wardens. They were to monitor collective dreaming, clandestine gatherings with an aim to form independent power bases and to control people who just never twigged on that the psychic community existed, of which there were some. Bazza trusted his new team. Although this was a full time job for him his team were volunteers, but with the responsibility that came with the position they also had privileged influence.

It was a bureaucratic blitzkrieg, it was established in a week and after three weeks people had accepted it. It was said to be necessary and propaganda was sent out, it was said that the movement was to combat Pete and people like him, who it was said had been in the process of revolution, Pete's end game was to form a satanic state. Street wardens and the like were there for the common good.

Other cities watched, Nicola had talked to them and told them that a "Pete incident" was waiting to happen in their city. She offered their councils the opportunity of visiting her city on fact finding missions. People in the city who did not like the movement turned to Pete and hoped for silent resistance groups.

"We need you Pete, we need you to fix this." was the rallying cry. Though Nicola too knew this was going on and it fed her paranoia. She told the council so much, they told her Pete was defeated and in time he'd be buried. After all he had not challenged them, yet.

Kelsang too was beginning to ponder that the city was turning into a People's Republic, he'd seen it happen in Tibet, and there his people had lost. He'd escaped these crazy social engineers.

He'd been spoken to by a street warden, a Mister Hartnet. The conversation had gone as follows;

"Ah Kelsang I believe, my name is Hartnet, I am the new warden. I think you'll fit in brilliantly, our street are a friendly lot. I think it would be splendid if you could show some of your wisdom, I am trying to set up a surgery in the Collins Community, I'll have to send it upstairs to get the okay but maybe you could represent some of our ethnic neighbours." Kelsang had put his hands together in a prayer position and bowed;

"I work at the centre too, I am sure it won't be a problem." he replied cordially. Mr Hartnet did not know what to say, he knew of Kelsang's association with the renegades. Kelsang knew he knew this but he pretended he thought that their talk was finished, and backed off and closed the door leaving the warden standing outside. Apart from his dislike of the warden he had Alex inside. Although Alex was not on one of the top suppressive individual lists he was still on it. So as Kelsang had seen this before, he wasn't going to send him away and a low profile was going to be paramount. He knew he'd be getting a knock on the door sooner or later asking loaded questions, and trying to frustrate his life. But although he would not personally aggravate the authorities he would fight if they tried to bring him down. Many of his fellow monks had suffered prison and were living in ghastly conditions. It was a delicate situation, how would he stop this terrible business happening here?

"One of those nosy wardens" he said to Alex.

"Were they looking for me?"

"Oh no, not at all, just trying to see whose side I was on."

"My parents are worrying, they sense the recent changes of power and are trying to live with it, they are in two minds as to whether it's a good thing, they're all talking about residents' meetings and the like. They say they are going to take part." Kelsang did not comfort him, he saw it would be more profitable for Alex to come to his own conclusion.

"Sit down and think about it, I will send you some protection for the while." He'd walked to the east in the early hours of the previous night, when going to Kelsang's he no longer took public transport, surveillance was a big thing now, it was safer to walk. Kelsang was emotional, he spoke;

"They will probably start bringing people in, people they think they can break, figures who they believe people look up to. For detention. For enforcement. For show trails." For the first time Alex thought Kelsang looked animated, ghosts of the past he guessed, he hoped these ghosts stayed in the past.

"Man it will be all right." Alex knew if he was with him he'd be all right. But then how did he know? Kelsang was a great person, he had saved Pete, Alex thought him superhuman. A glowing light in a (as he saw it) now dying continent. No, nothing could harm Kelsang. He sat back on the cushion where Kelsang had told him to sit the first time he was in the house. He thought things over, and thought through the evening and into the night, Kelsang sitting opposite him.

Chapter 42
An Escape to Where?

Pete thought the new goings on funny. He sat in his house watching television he had picked up in a thrift shop. At least they had not doctored the programmes on television, yet. He noticed now when he set out about a quarter of the people he passed gave him funny looks and whispered. It did not bother Pete, he chuckled;

"You can't hide genius," though he admired it; these passers by did not. It made Jackie and her team worry about him, Alex respected it and Joe Bob thought it funny. Joe Bob thought he had the same thing, though he was less willing to publicise it, his family had always acknowledged it but disapprovingly. Joe Bob kept his feelings about that time private. It had been quite a step escaping that lifestyle, he had seen psychology being used for evil. His phantoms were now mental health workers, they tried the same but he could handle them because he now had space away from family and "childhood friends"- Pete was his friend.

Pete snapped out of his reminiscences, the television was boring him. He'd moved to the west to escape certain types of people, now they seemed to be flooding the area. There had been an unusual amount of new people moving into the district - five in the last week, and they did not fit in but the residents welcomed them with a dread of what they brought. Wolfie had kept him up to date with this centralised fascist led revolt. These new people were part of that, he came to the conclusion he should just ignore them. But then before this all took place, when it was only the organization against him, Kelsangs's words came back to him;

"Give them a reason." "Give them a reason." he repeated it to himself. He did not know what action Kelsang had been referring to. He stood up and left for Joe Bob's. Not so many of the residents in the west welcomed Nicola's psychic revolution, they had been involved in shady goings on themselves, when Pete walked past they cursed him under their breath, it was all Pete's fault this was happening. They were pissed off.

Pete walked the whole way to the south, in the west he was edgy as hell but once he got to the south he calmed down a bit. He walked down an avenue of pollarded trees and houses with high hedges and long driveways. It was a different pace of life here to the west, here were wealthy families whose children all went to private schools. It was half eight in the evening and television light seeped out from windows of darkened sitting rooms. Pete wished he was in their situation, a nice family and privacy, people who responded to you with returned love.

Lost in his thoughts he arrived at the hostel door. He rapped the knocker and was left waiting for a long minute. Then he saw Padraic through the glass, the door opened, but he did not invite Pete in.

"Hello" said Pete.

"Hello" replied Padraic. He stood in Pete's way.

"Are the guys in?"

"Yes." He looked at Pete with a disparaging stare. But then Joe Bob pushed past him and patted Pete on the shoulder with fondness for his pal. They began to chat and Padraic stood behind them, they continued and after a bit he turned away and went to the office. The guys could hear him grumbling to Olivia. Joe Bob went close to Pete and whispered,

"Come on over to the Golden Horse." Joe Bob slipped out, taking care to close the door quietly, he should not have to do this, he told himself. Pete got the formalities out of the way;

"What will it be?"

"Whisky." Pete was going to say his order to the barman when the barman asked,

"How are things? Keeping well?"

"How unfortunate one person could create so much" he told himself.

"Yes." They both smiled and Pete got the whisky and half a stout for himself. Pete said,

"So how are you handling things?" Joe Bob was silent; he was collecting his thoughts. Pete had never seen him like this. He became white and when he spoke he spoke quickly,

"The organization have brought out a new policy, they want to keep us "the mental health service users" out of the community in a project out of town. Of course Padraic's trying to push us into it, all this fucking bullshit."

"Shit man" Pete blurted out. Joe Bob continued.

"It's strict 24 hour support, but it's really a segregated community with overseers and compulsory activities, and we're also only allowed out on "field trips"" The whole thing sounded shitty to Pete.

"When is all this happening?"

"It'll take a while, but Padraic's already making plans to stay top dog. It's all politics. Can I stay with you?" Pete was at war and this surprised him but he said,

"Yeah, sure." Joe Bob was a friend and one could still keep a bit of a low profile in the west district, he doubted they'd send the police looking for Joe Bob. At least not until the government was established. It was all go now; the web had been spun.

So they made a plan of escape. Now was the time. So Pete waited in the bar for half an hour while Joe Bob got his stuff, then he sneaked into the hostel garden and tapped Joe Bob's window, Joe Bob passed his rucksack of processions, clothes and stuff and then Pete walked down the road and they were soon on their way. Joe Bob had crept past the office and so he had escaped. They felt like he'd just got away with something like a bank robbery.

They strode down the road. Pete did not bother to hide, he just knew they'd get to his house okay and they did. Pete thought the area's bad perilous atmosphere would mess Joe Bob's mood but it did not. Pete saw that Joe Bob was not fazed and that meant he could concentrate, he hoped Joe Bob would help Pete with his plans but he'd be okay if he did not.

A neighbour who Pete had never met but who, unknown to Pete, had been watching him watched him and his new friend enter the house. She sat back down on her chair and turned back to the soap opera, and thought,

"The outside may have gone to shit but I've still got my soap operas." She glugged some warm tea and thought again,

"How could that scrawny guy have screwed things up so much?" She was a lonely old woman who had little contact with society but she was still an avid viewer of city 29's politics, though recently it had begun to worry her, but who was she?

Pete hauled up Joe Bob's bags into a spare room, it had no furniture but then Pete hadn't been expecting anyone. He would go into town tomorrow and get an inflatable bed for him to lie on and a sleeping bag to keep him warm. Downstairs Joe Bob had made himself at home, Pete broke out some tobacco and they watched the local news. How out of sync it was, physical crime was not the problem, it was society's psychic evil that was, that was never on the news.

The two of them stayed up all night. Joe Bob thought these clampets at the hostel would probably be looking for him, they'd phone his doctor tomorrow, he knew that the official police line would be that he was an adult, he was not missing, after all he'd taken his stuff with him, but it would filter up to the organization, would they do anything? Neither of them knew. Screw the lot of them, Padraic, his doctor, his foster parents, fuck the lot of them. Joe Bob smoked tobacco and swigged down tea and got used to his new found privacy. He laughed. Pete was glad he could accommodate his friend.

Chapter 43
Fighting from the Living Room

Jackie was having trouble with these "assholes" (as she called them). Her husband was working harder trying for solstice and home life had become ice cold. He was not really involved in anything, he enjoyed life in the rugby club and mammoth drinking sessions with his pals. Him and his mates had decided in high school to leave all the psychic business to the clever people, they were left alone to have a good time. But his wife was on some sort of hit list and some party official at work had treated him like he had made some foolish mistake and needed to be helped. He struggled to stop cracking up, if he so much as raised an eyebrow to the official she would not give him a "second chance." His Jackie had it easy, she did not work, she was free to play with her funny friends. He came home from work each day and Jackie did her best to make him forget with comfort food and hot sex, she really did her best.

After being home a couple of hours she called to her husband that she was leaving for her friends, Julius and Mary.

"No you're not, I don't want you to go, I can't, I mean all this trouble I've had and you still..." he began to moan and cry to her,

"Come back!" She turned to him, walked over to him and sat down.

"I'll get you help, we have to fight against this oppression, you and your rugby mates will soon be assimilated into this fascism, you understand, I'll sort something out tonight, it will be easier I promise." She left him sobbing.

She drove away, tears ran down her face as she swerved around a man crossing the road, he shook his fist at her. Five minutes later she made it to Julius's house. She walked to the door and saw Mary looking out of the window, she had a frown on her face. Julius opened the door, he lived in a roomy bungalow on his own but tonight he was also minding his eight year old nephew. Jackie followed him in and he called to the nephew,

"Get that homework done, your uncle and his friends need to talk, I'll check it in half an hour, and keep that television off."

They gathered. Mary told her guides to keep an aura of peace and began the proceedings. All of them wanted to speak. Julius said calmly,

"My relatives say this is beginning to remind them of China in the seventies." Jackie replied,

"My husband's having trouble at work, I said you'd help him Mary."

"Okay, okay we will help ourselves first then we will continue with our proper affair. Okay Jackie, I will send a band of ghosts sympathetic to us to help your Leo. Hopefully scare off anyone who tries to give him a hard time. I'll get them to go home with you and you can introduce them to him, best not to give him a fright."

Jackie looked round in the ether, in the spirit world, she could see a troupe of peculiar people, there was a guy in a denim jacket, a guy in a pin striped suit smoking a cigarette and about seven others, they did not seem that bothered, they looked capable but casual.

"You can talk to them later, we need to get down to business" urged Mary. Julius lost his temper, and swore,

"Business? The whole city 29 has gone to shit, possibly the whole world, us, three low lives and Pete - some Mahatma Gandhi want to be? We have enough trouble protecting ourselves. Andy did the right thing, he left our group when he could, and what's more is that that dratted Heathcliffe keeps coming over to me saying he has the whole spirit world behind him and to give up!"

Mary was the only one in the room keeping her cool. She spoke in a calm and controlled way;

"Now that's not true." She laughed, though there was a trace of panic there.

"No, I know for a fact that the spirits' world will always carry on as it has from the start of time and when the eight die their power won't transfer with them. Now, come on, what can we do?" she rallied.

"Well we need to tell people that in reality the eight and our former church have no mandate on them" said Jackie, she'd surprised herself but Julius countered,

"Who are we going to tell? They have the town captured, no one's gonna rise up against them. Physically and psychically we can't do shit."

"I think," said Mary, "that for now we have to protect ourselves and our loved ones. Leave Pete he will look after himself, we can only wait and hopefully the new ruling organization will fall in on itself. They can only attack us on one plain, the physical plain. Our minds are free and this is what we have to promote - mind freedom."

She stopped talking. Julius was lost in thought, for a second he thought her plan might work, then he muttered and spoke.

"That does not change anything, the fact is that someone has to end this tyranny. What if this is only the start and some epidemic spreads through the whole world, permeating into the peaceful tolerant life we have always known? No, if we take no action that could make the difference, everyone who cares for freedom has to try. We have to attack, no Queensbury rules."

Jackie was brave, although she was a woman she could be quite pugnacious, her Leo was the same. She improvised;

"We curse these Wardens, they are the weak link in the chain, a jumped up motley crew of office workers from the north. They think power comes with the job not the person, we attack." She stopped and hoped someone would continue her brainstorming. Mary spoke to Julius;

"Okay, what do you think?" He shrugged his shoulders,

"Yeah, I suppose." It was on, the three were going to fight, fight the good fight. This would take regular activity, they'd need to keep up any pressure they exerted. How to attack? They would do it like Che Guevara, quick attacks with maximum damage, then hasty retreats. This would hopefully make their presence known and the plan was that the populous would be so fed up that gradually they'd build up support, support that would then instigate attacks too.

The Priest had been tracking them He had a smile on his face. The group already had extra support and they did not know it.

Chapter 44
A Meeting, the First of Many?

The secret eight that had successfully regulated life before the Nile incident had changed to a secret twenty one. There was not much room in the conference room. The military installation had become a focal point of new urban development. There were even a couple of observers from other cities as well as a friend of Saul's from French Africa, she was staying at his house and had great influence back home. Saul now chaired, Nicola was now president and now officially overseer of the city, a puffed up mayor.

She and Saul were at the head of the table, she was in control. As Saul called for quiet and read out the agenda she was thinking. People began giving reports from their districts, Bazza and Connor sat amongst them, their loyalty had rewarded them. Carson smirked. These two both sat with designer suits on. Carson disliked this new rabble that Nicola had brought in, the new members were so eager to make a name for themselves that Carson felt a lot of important things were being overlooked, they had little experience. One of them were talking now;

"…and in conclusion the headmaster of the local school has let us have bi monthly meetings with the staff." Before the next person began, Nicola stood up;

"I think this is a splendid idea, all of you ought to do the same, the young are important, they will be our proud followers and new workers of our future metropolis. Carry on, thank you." Bazza spoke, he stood and shuffled his feet nervously;

"I think we should use internment, detention for those who wish to harm our government. I am thinking of Pete…" Interruption.

"And Jackie." Everyone was getting pissed off with that box, but Nicola always said they needed key members of the spirit world to have an input. Curtly she replied,

"No Bazza, we have to keep a constitution of sorts, we don't need a martyr or rebellion, but I propose we bring in some voodoo doctors in the meanwhile. Saul, you do that, scary people you can handle and the scarier the better, Bazza is right in that respect, we need a bit of terror. What was it Mao said? Barrel of the gun and all that." The rest of the meeting consisted of area heads doing battle with each other to impress their employers the most. Some things said were;

"We need to teach our wards to be patriotic."

"Some children should be told to make us aware of parental deviance."

"We need to stamp out cannabis use, it's making the teens think."

"I think we should use phone taps and listening devices." The last one raised a few eyebrows. Carson tried to gather the ideas into some coherence;

"Yes good, from what I've heard we need propaganda, we need some intelligence squad set up to plant listening devices, monitor emails, yes good work everyone." Nicola nudged Saul. He looked at his watch and said,

"Oh yeah, time, okay everyone, good stuff, you've all done well, could the "a" team stay behind." Thirteen people filed out, a couple hung back uneasy at the obvious segregation of power. Nicola stared at them with a forced grin on her face. They left.

"Any other business?" she asked, now ignoring Saul's chair.

"What are you doing about Pete?" This came from Curtis who more often gave advice rather than made policies. Nicola sucked on her finger and said,

"Establishing our works is more important, leave him to Saul's voodoo doctors to sort him out." Saul looked around unsure, he was used to people like the Professor but these voodoo doctors were on another level, these guys were weird, they lived life between worlds, they'd have strange demands and manners. Although most lived in Africa there were some in Europe, he had heard a rumour that some were used in the second world war by both sides, but it had been a long time since they'd been employed by any government; they should have employed Pete, he thought ironically.

He'd ask the spiritualists for help here. His thinking was that it was strange for a living person to become a voodoo doctor, at least in Europe, therefore the spiritualist ghosts were bound to have heard or run in with someone like the one they needed, so he said,

"I think we should leave it to Heathcliffe to get the help we need."

"I think we should be careful, look what happened last time we brought in outside help." This was Curtis speaking.

"Well yes, I guess so. But let's not completely dismiss it"

said Nicola. Saul was kind of relieved, he didn't like spooky people.

"Controlled religion." It was that damn box again, Saul and a couple of the others thought. Though Nicola told it,

"Go on." The box coughed a couple of times, clearing its throat.

"The people need church, moral guidance in our new utopia for the masses, and I urge you to use my church, make it a church that will last an eternity, one based on our enlightened society that will transcend death." This really blew the eight away. Carson spluttered that this was exactly the kind of shit that the masses might buy.

"By Jove, you're right, yes this is something we need. Save the people on two fronts, watched by the wardens developed by the church. Yes." Saul wasn't religious and thought all religion was social control, but if people were stupid it was up to them. He disliked the way this new movement was going, he'd liked it pre Nile. People were generally free to think and associate, they'd only been there to stop crazy renegades but he was not going to leave. Carson took the lead,

"Okay Heathcliffe my friend, we'll sort out a meeting at your church." Heathcliffe flew away to tell Oliver and the others what had just happened. They had discussed a new wave church but nobody back at that church in the south had expected the idea to go down so well.

Chapter 45
Insurgencies

Alex was moping about Kelsang's house. Kelsang was annoyed and told him to wise up and snap out of it. Kelsang snapped,

"All these things happening are external, you should still be at home in your mind, I am and I used to live in Tibet. Come sit with me." The room had a thin smoke of incense sticks and Kelsang picked up a singing bowl (made of copper, used for meditation) which when he hit it gave a deep ring. They sat opposite Kelsang meditating and Alex tried to follow the lead but he couldn't. After ten minutes he stood up and looked down on Alex who was in the lotus position. He said,

"Okay, okay Alex we'll do something. I never liked that Hartnet guy, perhaps we can start on him." Clapping his hands Alex said,

"Good good." They went to the room at the top of the house, it was not used often although it was kept clean and free from dust. It also had cushions. They sat down, it did not have a light bulb and it was getting dark outside. Klesang mumbled in his native tongue. Alex wondered how anyone could decipher that peculiar sound (the native Tibetan tongue). Then for his benefit English was spoken.

"We call on spirits of mischief to look in on our friend Mr Hartnet, may you make his job of warden hard and fickle, though let no violence befall our friend. May his friends and colleagues joke about him and may he not hear it, may women see his body naked, may his superiors not hear his problems." Alex chipped in,

"When he dreams may he think himself a woman."

"And may this all come true as it is in your world." Alex giggled, his mind had forgotten about his troubles for now and felt that at least they'd done something, they went back downstairs and Alex began to cook some toast with boiled eggs, he liked the eggs nice and runny.

The next morning they left the house for a walk, even though Alex was meant to be keeping a low profile. City 29 was bathed in a cold sun. There was a queer merriment with the people of the east district, they seemed to ignore the man in orange robes and the young fellow following him. The two stopped at a bakery and bought an éclair bun each, they continued to the Collins community centre licking cream from their lips. They walked in to the office that Sadie, a neighbour from a couple of streets away used to work in. She was used to being in charge before Hartnet had come along.

She was there trying to retain some normality, she looked up and said,

"We weren't expecting you today, some of the kids have been having a bit of trouble recently, in school. Would you talk to them?"

"I thought this was Hartnet's office, where is he today?"

"Oh, he's walking about here somewhere." This was followed by a titter. Alex raised an eyebrow and they did not have to wait long until they bumped into him.

"Why, Mr Hartnet."

"Oh, hello." He seemed uncomfortable and kept stroking his leg. Sadie and another worker stood behind him giggling.

"I am a tail wagging bitch dog" he blurted out. Kelsang put out his hand and opened and closed his fist.

"You will go home and think twice about wielding such power, you will help the people." He turned and walked away unmindful of the community laughing at him. Sadie stood beside Kelsang and mentioned,

"That horrible man was like that all this morning, he went and said to me he liked my dress and that it brought out my eyes then he came out as a homosexual. I don't know what's going on, I guess if you do bad it catches up on you. I'll confide in you Kelsang because I know you are not one of them, this community has had its heart ripped out in these past days and he and his sort are the culprits. It's the same in all the districts, not only the east side, my sister from the west, she…" A queer chatterbox Kelsang thought, he nodded as she spoke, Alex was fiddling about with the vending machine. It threw out a cola when he wanted a lemonade.

Kelsang came to his side. He walked Alex with him to the games room where the disobedient children were playing. They ran up to him and he patted them on the shoulder.

"Okay, okay now what's the problem boys?" A small boy who Kelsang knew to be happy and to enjoy his young life began;

"We were in class with Mrs Good and the new school councillor sat at the back. She told Mrs Good that she was "not up to scratch" and when I defended her and told that old bat to shut up she looked at me and my friend and I was shaking the rest of the day and my mummy was all worried."

"Okay." He put his hand back on the boy's shoulder and said, "Don't worry, it's okay." The boys thought for a bit and then they could see who they could trust in the world and who they couldn't; strange. Alex asked one of them for a game of pool and they got back to playtime.

Meanwhile Pete woke up Joe Bob and they drank coffee and ate digestive biscuits. They watched the local news, no mention of Joe Bob the escapee. Pete imagined that back at the hostel Dwight would be asking where Joe Bob was and Padraic would have noticed that all his clothes were gone and perhaps he thought he might be in trouble, he'd have to report this to the warden, it wouldn't look good. Pete wondered if anyone else would miss Joe Bob. Pete had never asked him about family, but neither had he asked Pete. What to do today?

"Any ideas what to do today, Joe Bob?" He was surprised by the answer.

"Let's visit Voodoo man, he lives nearby doesn't he?"

"Yep, three streets away." Indifferent, they set off. People stared at them; when they arrived and knocked Voodoo man's door, a neighbour peeked through the blinds. Voodoo man's door opened. And there he was. Last time he'd met Voodoo man he had been gaunt and pale and then when he had made eye contact he'd had a look of trepidation, but now he seemed cool and easy going, but Pete could tell he was still involved in the ongoing power struggle. Joe Bob said,

"Hey man what's happening?"

"Not much, I guess you guys can come in." They followed him in, the house was the same as Pete's though it was better furnished, he had a new sofa and a couple a prints of ocean sunsets, also it had been newly decorated. Pete thought his father the Professor had probably taken him out and got all this stuff now they were talking again. Joe Bob continued,

"So what do you think about all this shit?"

"What shit?"

"You know, all this totalitarian bullshit."

"Doesn't bother me, I lead my own life, those new orders and stuff, fucked if I care." Pete expected this, but who was he to make a judgement?

"You and Pete were involved with that demon Nile. It was

him that started this order, don't you think it's messed up?"

"That's more dad's business than mine" Joe Bob prodded him.

"But can we count on you to help hammer them to the ground?" Voodoo man looked Joe Bob in the eye, was he trying to stare him out or was he thinking about it? Pete did not know. Voodoo man kept staring at him and Joe Bob stared back, then Voodoo man's eyes lit up and he sent a vibe to Joe Bob, it was loud and Pete felt it, it said,

"I'll help you out no problem if I am round your way." This was more than Pete expected, they joined together in their collective minds and gave a high five then they were back in the room, Wolfie came in, he'd missed the high five. He had something to say.

Pete looked at him and showed solidarity with the three of them. Wolfie raised his eyebrows with a look of doubt but Pete said,

"Yes." Then Pete noticed Voodoo man was watching him. Pete said,

"It's all right, he's a pal of mine." Voodoo man did not care if he was a friend or not, he didn't like his affairs being told to people he didn't know, but he let it go giving Pete a dirty look. Joe Bob talked.

"Listen man, we don't do anything too proactive, we basically just hang out and see what happens, kinda keep it in the comfort zone if you know what I mean."

Voodoo man was beginning to like these two cats. He lay back and broke out some tobacco and turned on the television which he did not often watch. Wolfie wanted to talk, he talked out of Pete's mouth so they could all hear,

"It's terrible, it seems that the organization are setting up their own religion, they think they're setting up a fourth Reich or something. They're going to use the Spiritualist Church as the power base under the guise of some new creed, it's got full support from the eight which by the way is now the twenty one." He paused for effect, but Pete spoke,

"Well guys the solution is simple, we start our own religion." He thought for a second, the guys looked curious which was good, he continued,

"We make it fun, we make it psychic friendship, our own psychic church." Joe Bob and Voodoo man liked it, Wolfie thought it damn dangerous. Voodoo man said,

"Yeah, we'll be the leaders, I know what's good, what we should provide."

"Yeah, we'll start our own community" Joe Bob said. Pete was a bit worried that they did not recognize the danger of this, it was declaring war. Maybe those two had always been at war to some extent. Pete thought,

"Wolfie can rally up some support on his side." Wolfie did not say anything but Pete knew Wolfie was on board. Pete went for it -

"Well let's start now." They all seemed to know what to do, they stood in Voodoo man's lounge, together, and held hands, they sent out the invitation to all sentient beings in city 29. It showed the reward of joining together and also the immediate need of joining together, it had the power of an atom bomb and went out like its wave, everyone in the whole city heard and tuned in. The whole city also saw who had sent it. Would they join? Many of them would. The war was on.

Chapter 46
Shockwave

As the bomb went off Jackie was sitting with Leo, he was more at ease now the spirits of Mary were around, he was becoming quite accomplished himself now, their ways were rubbing off on him and Jackie reflected he was becoming quite powerful. She was happy. The bomb went off and Jackie spilt her coffee over her lap.

"Shit!" she exclaimed. Leo raised his eyebrows.

"That's Pete." he said. "Was that a message to us, or did others hear it? He's starting something and I am up for it."

"Me too. I am going to phone Mary." It was a bit pointless she already knew, she could see her ghost friends and Leo's protectors were equally shaken.

"Hello, Mary?" There was a cackle of laughter on the other side of the line, then speaking quickly Mary said,

"Ha ha, yes I heard them, this is what we've been waiting for, I am joining immediately, see you there. You coming with me?" She meant in an astral way.

There was sort of traffic, a tail back. The three received them all and they stood together, they stood all of them, free, giving out their own vibes, vibes of love, vibes hinting at the surrealism of the situation. Finally they could do what they pleased in this heavily policed plain, and it was Pete, Joe Bob and Voodoo man who were responsible.

The people who had given Pete dirty looks now surrounded him, the kids at the Collins Community flocked, their parents following, wandering aimlessly in the streets. Joe Bob and Voodoo man welcomed them, ushering all the people into their mind. Even the Priest was there, all the ghosts in the city, although those not under the tyranny clapped and yelled. The Professor patted his son on the back. Even Saul felt the righteousness and power but he hung back. Had he left he felt he could have been seen as some sort of hypocrite, he hung back for now. His phone rang.

Kelsang and Alex also hung back and watched how the city 29's karma changed and morphed. Had this happened in Tibet they would have been crushed by the authorities, Kelsang reflected. But he couldn't refrain from smiling at the plethora of people travelling away from the organization's recent oppression. And it was all happening in Voodoo man's small terraced house in the west.

Pete and the others laughed at their achievement. There were over a thousand souls in their psychic gathering. Pete although silent physically was shouting at the top of his voice mentally. The three stood up and began walking the streets. People saw them from their front rooms and cheered, as they walked passed people the people stopped and watched them walk away, witnessing this majestic happening.

The three stopped and again held hands, music came out of their minds, trance like music with pumping drums, the hundreds of people who'd gathered with them could hear it and they also brought their friends. Everyone listened,

"A new age has come" someone proclaimed. Pete, Voodoo man and Joe Bob continued walking, they kept putting in new mixes and speeding it up and adding vocals, it was beautiful. More and more people joined them. Even people in far away lands could detect the wave of change occurring in Pete's city.

Nicola had felt the bomb as well and all the twenty one minus a causality from the east district (Hartnet) had gathered half an hour after it. Nicola ignored Saul's position as chair and tried to make her speech sound less like a rant, but she was shaking.

"I didn't expect this, we are experiencing a revolution, and if it spreads we are all in trouble." A couple of members were tapping their feet and drumming on the conference room's table, they couldn't ignore the funky beats, Nicola ignored them and the music only made her angry.

"Physical action alas has now become necessary, Bazza and Connor, take an interceptor car, track them down by following the music, take them alive and bring them back to the detention centre in the installation."

"Detention centre?"

"We have prepared for such an event and yes we have a detention centre, go to building A-5." Bazza and Connor left and went to the garage; they also armed themselves with taser guns, truncheons and a couple of Glock 7 revolvers. Even though they were not meant to kill them, they could still shoot them in the leg if needed, maybe the threat of the guns would work.

They got in the car, it was unmarked but did have flashing blue lights from the radiator and a siren could be put on the roof if needed. It was ten times better than that old blue sierra. He floored it and flew down the main carriage way to the centre of the city, then onto the streets of the west. They listened to the music and could see all the citizens swarming around it. People stood at their front doors together, united and dancing ecstatically. Connor understood why they had to be stopped. And there they were "walking like swaggering cowboys", Bazza thought. He hit the sirens. Pete looked round; they ran away into a local park. Bazza and Connor got out of the car.

Pete looked around, these were the guys from the blue sierra who'd started on him the other day. He said,

"Keep the music guys, and run." Joe Bob and Voodoo man turned around and saw the two plain clothes police running at them. Pete fancied himself as an MC and as he ran he broke into the music that the others kept going and began to say,

"Respect the west, respect the east, respect the south and the hostel, this is MC Pete to say your psychic radio is under threat but to keep listening." The music blared and Bazza tried to ignore it to make his job easier but Connor couldn't stop, he was finding it hard.

The guys generated it into house music and vaulted over a wall into a play ground. A group of youths sat on the swings having a smoke of spliff and cheered with celebration as the three sprinted past. The two following were yelled at but that didn't matter, they got over the wall too. They were now running down to a car park, but had reached a dead end. Shit. Pete, Joe Bob and Voodoo man turned and looked Connor and Bazza in the eyes. The music was pulsing through Bazza and Connor as they were so close to these three generators. Bazza got out his walkie talkie.

"Fox trot twenty one five delta this is hero we have the suspects at the car park of Glen road. Please advise." There was white noise and for a second he thought these psychic disc jockeys had affected their radio, but it buzzed back.

"We are sending a car hero, this is fox trot twenty one delta. Out."

Voodoo man ran at Connor but was zapped by the taser gun and hit the ground convulsing. But Pete and Joe Bob stayed still, they did not fear or care about being caught. Pete murmured to Joe Bob;

"It would be a strange trip getting arrested." They cuffed Voodoo man and showed Pete and Joe Bob their guns. Pete and Joe Bob hung back. Pete slowed the music down and began to smoke a rollie he had already made. Connor, amazed they'd caught these

enemies, spluttered,
"Put that out."
"Fuck off."

Chapter 47
Immediate Aftermath

One hour later at a special meeting at the installation the twenty strong organization and the eight spiritualists lead by Eugene were having a sit down. Five minutes ago the music had stopped abruptly. Carson had nominated himself to listen in on the music in case they gave anything away, what sort of things he did not know. But Pete had given the populous a step by step account of their arrest and where they'd been taken to and had even kept a bass line going although it had gone quite experimental.

They'd been taken to the detention centre which was near the clinic Nicola had recovered in after she had been attacked by Nile. The guards had picked them up in an estate car with blacked out windows and had injected each of them with a sedative to stop the telepathic dance. It worked immediately on Voodoo man but Pete and Joe Bob resisted it in the mind but it did semi paralyse them. They'd then been carried into individual cells in a hidden wing of the installation that was underground. The cells were reinforced by a magnetic force field that was able contain their psychic radio. The hundreds of people just heard it go dead, the last thing was Joe Bob saying,

"We are underground in the military installation in the north and they are putting us into strange metallic rooms." Then nothing. Nicola was relieved. Saul spoke;

"Well as you perhaps have realised, we have them contained. We have a lot of work to do, we'll never be trusted by certain sections of our city again. We need to still cater for every citizen's needs, to protect them, and to help them." He paused, there were coughs of approval.

"We need to satisfy them spiritually, if we can learn one thing from this sorry incident it is that."

"We need to interrogate them and find the truth." It was Carson.

"Don't you worry, tell the masses we are keeping them for protection, and that some satanic cult is jealous, and is after them. Yeah, that will be the cover story, but we will be imposing on them a strict regime around the clock, they will regret this day's activity. I have some people stepping in, trained by our brothers in China. Things will be normal soon, with censorship, monitoring of the

Internet; people will forget."

Nicola slouched back into her seat; why should she do it all? Back to Saul.

"Okay, we also need to *normalise* psychic activity, that's where our friends from the spiritualist church will help." He stopped and the room turned its attention on Eugene.

"It seems with the infinite masses of the universe we will always be outnumbered in the world of the dead. We have to go to the people and move them physically and mentally. They will follow. They were only active for two hours and a quarter. Maybe we could get one of our own to be the "new officially endorsed" Pete." That's what Eugene thought. Then Curtis spoke, as he rarely did none of the new members knew who he was.

"What about the Voodoo Doctors, the Voodoo science people Saul was meant to get? Surely fear would help our rule." Saul countered,

"I will phone them now and tell them of our emergency, they'll be here tomorrow." Then Nicola spoke.

"Well Eugene, you and your friends are now part of our new think tank, but you will be supervised by Saul." Saul clenched his fist. Why should he be the one to entertain these idiot people? He looked at Iris who was present with her tattered woolly jumper.

Quite rightly Alex was worried, he had been listening and wished they'd texted him so he could have been a part of it. Kelsang had thought the music a racket and had just gone about his normal business of devotional meditation. Alex could not believe that, he'd asked Alex to make him his tea and Alex had lost his patience and said,

"I can't believe you, this is the greatest thing I've ever heard, how can you sit like that?" Kelsang looked at him, Alex felt a momentary horror at what he'd just done, he was the disciple. So he got up and made the tea. But he danced while he made it. But even this annoyed Kelsang; dance was a distraction from dwelling on the true nature of his mind. If Alex was a child he would have got a beating.

They sat together and Kelsang tried to explain a passive aggression.

"But I still love those guys."

"So do I. Try not to listen; be calm." And Alex was calm. They drank their tea, the mind hurricane outside. Kelsang did not try to distract him, he had to learn for himself. They sat for an hour, Alex did succeed in disassociating himself from what the rest of the city heard, he found himself happy and began to read some sutras Kelsang gave him, then suddenly Kelsang said to Alex,

"Listen, listen to Pete." He tuned in.

"....they are putting us into metallic rooms." Then nothing. Alex stood up. He panicked but Kelsang said,

"Not to worry, they have already done enough." They returned to their tea but Alex found it hard. The sight of the green steam put him in a dream - he was hovering in green steam and was looking down, he was with God and Pete's activity was a wave low down. It oscillated back and fourth in the world, there was a wave in the spirit world too but in his and Kelsang's world they were outside the wave's action on both sides. He returned to normality to see Kelsang watching him. He had his hands folded and he nodded his head.

"What to do about Pete?"

"He knows he's a wave and he knows how not to be a wave, he'll be back with us when he wants to." Alex couldn't accept that it, it was too cryptic. So he looked back and prayed for Pete. Alex said,

"Let's go to the centre."

"Okay, all right we'll go there." They ventured outside. It was like Christmas day as not many people were outside and those that were were kind of dazed. The community knew that the two of them were associated with Pete and Joe Bob, and they whispered as Alex and Kelsang walked past.

"Where are your friends?" asked a gaunt drug addict. Alex said,

"We only know as much as you, friend," and they strode on. And they made it to the centre. Still no Hartnett, but Sadie welcomed them in. She dived straight in,

"Is it going to last? Are we beaten before we started? Are you going to rescue them? How can we stop those wardens retaining their power?"

"We don't know, we only know as much as you." It was Alex talking.

Chapter 48
New Fronts are Drawn

Jackie did not like the music, she was from the eighties and was into country music. Her Leo tolerated that, most people hated country music. She had when it started liked the idea of the bomb, people together were great but as for that, what she thought was psychic vandalism they committed through their music, she thought it unnecessary. Now she was told by Julius on the phone that they had been caught and imprisoned in some force field room. She never wanted that.

The people who had joined in the revolt were hanging around thinking Pete would come back or something. The organization was beginning to rise again, something needed to be done. She phoned Mary and Julius and proposed an emergency meeting at his place. As she went out the door Leo shouted,

"I kind of liked the music, it reminded me of the summer of '89."

She drove to Julius's and kept one eye on the road and the other on the people still waiting about. She got to the bungalow and banged on the door and entered. Mary barged in after her and Jackie began immediately;

"We need to carry on the work that Pete and his friends started, we need to do it now, we need to send another bomb, those snakes at the installation have Pete and believe you me they'll already have started downplaying everything." The others let their approval be heard.

"Okay, everyone hold hands, let's send the bomb."

They held hands and sent out a wave. It was just as big as Pete's, the city felt it but it was a poor imitation. People just did not connect with it as they had Pete's. It said,

"Come people we need to work together, we need to stand as a new state." People just were not interested. So they returned their minds back to Julius's. He mumbled,

"Maybe we should bust Pete out." But the three of them knew this was silly. They watched as gradually people left, giving up on Pete returning for now, and went back to their business.

"How could the populous do this? They nearly had it" thought Jackie. The others began to think that fighting for ideals would not work, you had to really believe them then the people would believe in you. That's what Pete and his mates had, infectious belief, that's what scared the organization, and that's why they attacked Pete in the first place all those months ago. It would have saved a lot of bother had Pete been beaten then, but he just did not give up and now they had him interned.

The three sat around. Mary said,

"The only thing we can do is defend ourselves. When everyone else has gone down we shall still be here. That's all we can do."

"Okay, thanks for the ghosts you sent for my Leo, he's really getting into all the psychic stuff and probably won't even need them in a while. It's helped the marriage, he's all right about things that normally he used to dislike." Jackie spoke hastily.

They all started drinking teas and let the day's dust settle itself and watched as the wind blew it.

Across city 29 Saul's new focus group began the next day, his voodoo science friend had flown in from Ghana specially, another friend was also meant to come but had looked at everything and declined. Since yesterday's meeting the wardens had been debriefed, they'd been told to keep a check on the schools, churches and community centres and the like, to show control, to say they'd acknowledged the bomb and that they would be enforcing the good that came out of it but also that they would be correcting the wrong that Pete had brought by "mistake," and to top it off they said they were working with Pete for the good of the city.

Anyway the focus group began. Present were Saul, his African friend Tutu and the eight spiritualist elders, including Iris, Eugene and Oliver. The black box was also present, bringing Heathcliffe and Jeremiah to the meeting. They'd also with the help of Tutu put a barrier round the meeting to keep it private.

"We are gathered here at this think tank/focus group to create an official spiritual support for our citizens. Here to help us is a personal friend of mine, Tutu from Ghana, he is an expert in voodoo science. You think Pete's bomb was powerful? This guy can get a dislike for someone and "boom" he can make them *reconsider* their actions, this is where he can help us." Oliver spoke;

"Well we are here representing religion, we help people deal with death and promote good morals. We have decided to help to reinforce a good ethical standard."

"And I will help you, man." said Tutu in a thick African

accent that reminded Eugene of some poisoned charisma with a sinister undertone, but they carried on.

"Okay, this is good" said Saul, introducing optimism into the proceedings, then he said after a moment of contemplation,

"We need to regulate all this activity and only let it be done for the good of the collective. We need officials whose job is to be a gateway into any psychic activity, to build up an amicable mutual relationship, a new functionalist society. How do you think we can achieve this, Tutu?"

"Examples man, we make examples of people who went down the paths we do not like and if you allow me to bring in help maybe we could make Pete a new man and show him off to the people." Oliver then said,

"We need to recruit spirits and flood city 29 with these watchers who will be responsible to us and if any try and start anything then we leave it to Tutu and his friends."

"How long will this be, when will it be up and started?" asked Saul.

"We can have the spirits here in a day" said Oliver.

"I can make an example whenever you want" said Tutu.

"All right" said Saul, reading into Tutu's statement, "I have a file of all Pete's associates, I think the one to go for is the one called Dwight, a guy from his old hostel, he'd be the easiest. People will learn not to meddle in our social fabric."

Chapter 49
...Like a Ton of Bricks

Pete had been sitting on his ass all night on a tough styrofoam mattress. He could tell something was blinding his skills, so he'd stopped. The light was on all the time and the walls were made of Pyrex glass that gave out a blue light and a soft humming sound. There were eight cells and he could see Joe Bob and Voodoo man, but as well as being mind proof they were sound proof! They'd put him in an orange prison suit and given him a pair of flip flops, he'd also been given some cornflakes in a bowl with hardly any milk. Where they trying to break him?

He sat around all morning. He took a shit, it broke the time up and the others watched him, there was nothing to do. Around tea time two African guys stood outside the cells, Pete sent out a vibe but then he remembered it was blocked, one of them saw Pete's attempt and gave out a deep belly laugh but then Pete couldn't hear that either. He could only see the laugh. They smiled at him and walked off in deep conversation. Then at last something good happened.

"Psst." Pete looked around.

"Psst, it's Wolfie, friends listening in on the black box, this place is tight. See that big African gentleman? He's from the African federation of voodoo science. He's here to break you, Mocto says he's the real deal, everyone in Ghana knows him even if he doesn't know them. Just be careful, I'll be back." And Pete was alone. Over the next day and night various ghosts paid Pete visits, there was Alex's friend Mocto, the Priest. Now he was a laugh, he told him how they had the meeting and thought it all secret when a bunch of him and his pals were pissing themselves on the other side. So Pete did not feel so isolated, but was daunted about the future interrogation. Wolfie sent some sexy women ghosts and they massaged Pete and Voodoo man's shoulders with their own hands. Joe Bob declined. As this went on Pete sent some people over to his friends. Voodoo man had been worrying, his dad could not help, he needed his dad. He calmed down a bit with this company. Joe Bob did not need it. None of them blamed Pete; they were still together.

Pete was beginning to lose track of time; it was another morning, he thought. Bazza and Connor were outside, they had a microphone and Pete could hear what they said.

"Ah Pete, my friend, I just thought we'd pay my favourite deviant a visit." He twiddled about on a button on his jacket and said to the others,

"Oh and hello you two, you got involved with the wrong guy." They laughed, they had Pete where they wanted him and Pete couldn't do shit (in their view). Then they began to laugh even harder. Pete was bemused, then he blacked out.

"Gas Quetapine-25 always does the job" mumbled Bazza. A couple of heavies in nurses' smocks opened the door and hauled Pete out. When Pete woke up he was chained to a chair and he had some sort of neck brace on that stopped him moving his head. He felt a prick in his neck, he sent out a vibe to the people in the room but they did not react, the two Africans (Saul and Tutu) sat in front looking at him, the heavies stood behind, they had guns and other non lethal implements. Saul told him,

"Finally we meet, Pete. You may notice that you can't *look* the way you did, our helpful Chinese friends taught us to silence you. There is an acupuncture pin in your neck that does that exact job." Pete tried to wiggle his head but to no avail.

"We don't stand for your type where I come from, in Ghana they either join us or die." Pete felt shivers down his spine and began to shake in his seat.

"You will join me" Tutu continued. Saul felt his cause was being left out, what if Pete did join him, he'd told Nicola they would make an example of him, but what could he say? Although Tutu was a friend he had been wary of him, although he never said so. Since the request he'd been dreading bringing Tutu over because he knew he would not be accountable. He should not have boasted about his exotic acquaintances.

The way Tutu usually succeeded in cursing his country's renegades was to rely on them envying his collective, and that really messed up any psychic defence the renegades tried to put up, but Pete had no envy. He did not give a monkey's about some motley crew of voodoo practitioners, nor about their Ghana reputation that Wolfie had made him aware of. Yeah, this guy was the real McCoy but if you actually thought about it so what?

Tutu's eyes narrowed, he threw out a glare of playful hatred. Pete stopped himself returning a smile and luckily Tutu did not pick up on it. Saul spoke;

"You know Pete we can keep you here for as long as we want, we will keep you in that cell and gas you and interrogate you, gas you and interrogate as much as we want. Make it easy for yourself boy, sit in on our meetings and help us in our new world, eh? You have no real friends to let down, the two that came in here, they won't bother with you, you are all on different paths from them now." Pete did not even think about it, which was a mighty feat of disassociation from what was going on in itself. Tutu began to laugh, he laughed uncontrollably and Saul wanted to tell him to shut it. Tutu could not believe this guy, he'd never seen the like of it, this guy was an untouchable, he should have taken more notice, his other friend in Ghana had divined this but he'd been blind, he realised he'd come to witness the boy, he could not believe it.

But he had told Saul he'd do the job so he was stuck. He glinted to Saul's mind,

"We will get him just stay calm." Saul nodded to one of the heavies who injected Pete in the neck. They'd learnt he needed twice the normal dose. Pete was out. They wheeled him back to the cell and took the special acupuncture needle out.

Chapter 50
Awful Business

Dwight had been snatched. The organization goons had arrived at the hostel and Padraic had stood aside as they flashed their military IDs. They went to the smoking room and grabbed Dwight. As they pulled him out he screamed and Ryan had moved to help poor Dwight but he was pushed back and was not able to help. He called to Padraic to phone the police. He did not.

"Don't worry." a brutish goon sneered, "He'll be back, we are just taking him for help in our inquiries."

"They have Pete too" Ryan thought. He began to panic. Dwight was too vulnerable. These guys would tear him apart. He worried. Padraic entered the room;

"He must have got mixed up in something. You have to admit, Pete has gone too far." Ryan swore at him. Padraic turned his back on them and walked down to the office. As he left Danny shouted,

"Fucking cunt."

Dwight was being driven to the installation to building A-5 in one of the blacked out estate cars. He was sat in the middle with goons on either side. He was crying,

"You got the wrong man, you got the wrong man, it wasn't me." He cried more. The goons just looked ahead. Dwight began to shake, he grabbed one of the goon's arms,

"Please leave me, leave me home." He stopped crying and it became a sob.

They arrived at the installation gate and the guards did not stop the car, they just waved them through. Dwight looked out of the window, although it was blacked out he could make out the ominous buildings whose purpose he did not know.

They got to the covert detention centre Pete and the others were in and the heavies in white nurses' smocks came out and hauled Dwight inside. He yelled,

"You watch out, Pete will save me, yeah he'll get you." The goons raised an eyebrow. He'd stopped crying, but it was now partly shock. There was a reception with some bitch secretary who just smiled as they brought the distraught Dwight through.

They escorted him down corridors, then to the cells which were on an underground level. Dwight was put purposefully into a cell where Pete could see him. Pete was alarmed, but he gave a friendly wave in the hope it would appease any distress. Dwight surveyed the quarters. He began to look at the glass's blue glow and again began to panic,

"Pete, don't let them do anything to me." Pete held back tears, he could not hear his friend Dwight with the soundproof glass, he could not comfort him. Voodoo man and Joe Bob could not do anything, they just kept staring forward. They too had been gassed and interrogated, although Saul blamed Pete for everything. Right from the start when they had been forced to get Nile it was all Pete's fault, it was Pete that had caused them to seek Nile. They had tried to change Voodoo man, he was an inherent loner and was not interested in any deals, though Tutu had succeeded in torturing his mind. Saul had watched, how this torture worked was well over his head, he tried to learn but he could not pick it up, it was above him. It took a few hours but Voodoo man only recovered back in the cell.

Joe Bob was a different story, as soon as he snapped out of the quetipine gas Tutu was scared, when he leapt into Joe Bob's mind he saw indescribable torment, Joe Bob through millennia had lived with it. Tutu asked to tell him his story, he'd heard of these fallen angels although they were scarce. Joe Bob just looked ahead and glared, then when he looked at Tutu and showed him his fall and God's anger Tutu cried out.

"Shit" said Saul, "That needle, he can beat the jamming needle." Joe Bob looked away. Saul gasped, he looked round to see Tutu, he was on the ground having a convulsive fit. The heavies dashed forward and lifted Tutu into a chair. Saul held his head up, he was frightened, he could only see the whites of Tutu's eyes and he was jabbering away in someone else's voice.

"Get him away!" cried Saul, indicating Joe Bob. They hauled Joe Bob out back to the cell. Joe Bob did not betray what had gone on to his friends, he just lay on his bed, but he did look over to Dwight and gave the thumbs up.

Then they came for Dwight. For effect they did not bother to gas him, the heavies just took an arm each, ignored his panicked pleas and walked him to the interrogation room, then they strapped him into a chair. Tutu was sitting there, he was a bit more lucid but he was still in a cold sweat. He was still talking gibberish under his breath. Saul was there waiting for him.

"See what your friend did?" He walked over to Dwight and whacked him in the face. Then he turned and nodded and they helped Tutu up and he staggered away.

A nurse came and injected Dwight in the neck. Then he left.

Chapter 51
Imoonan Lands on Earth

In what was known as “The Travellers’ Airport Nevada” (it was over the size of greater London) Imoonan flew in, guiding the craft to the landing site. He landed and a car drove to the ship. The driver got out and met the space man. The man read the passport that entitled entrance to earth, you did not have to have one but it saved a lot of time, it was not the sort of planet that generally allowed sightseers. The passport was read,

“I cannot pronounce your name.”

“Im-oon-an. Im-oon-an is how it’s said.”

“Welcome, Imoonant. Your friend is waiting.” He did not bother to correct the way his name had been said. He got into the car and was driven to a customs centre. He had the atmos box of drugs in a rucksack. This world was steeped in corruption.

“Any sightings recently?” Imoonan made conversation. “Sightings” was a pejorative term; “leaks” would have been a more accurate word.

“Yeah, a bunch of Zalks flew over Mexico city on the day of the dead festival, their craft was seen by thousands.” Imoonan thought the guy wasn’t very talkative. Arriving, they walked quickly and Imoonan fell behind a bit.

“Hurry up.” They walked down a maze of corridors, past offices and clearing centres to a deserted café. The pharmaceutical agent was there with a cup of coffee.

“I’ll leave you guys.” Imoonan walked towards the agent, this was well dodgy business but there was no way he’d be done/prosecuted by anyone, clandestine deals like Imoonan‘s happened every week on this planet.

“Your Rock-too leaves. Hard to come by, you got the greens?” He was handed a brown envelope with crisp dollar bills in return for the atmos box.

“Thank you,” and that was the deal completed.

“Any other business, give me a phone.” offered the agent.

“Yeah, no bother.” He probably would not get the chance to phone as this was a deal of a life time. The agent had opened the box and was rubbing one of the leaves in his hand, smelling the oil of the leaf.

He wondered about the other illicit drugs he knew and if

they‘d be interested. He was sure that the pharmaceutical company in all probability knew more about inter planetary drugs than he did. But he had the phone, it did not work in deep space but it worked in trading planets. Imoonan had had it modified, he had infinite credit and he could tune it in on planets to access their telecommunication systems.

He phoned his sister, but her phone was not active. He left a message, he did not like family poking their noses into his business but they were blood and had useful connections. When with them he'd bump into some old Mayan friends and that was good.

He left the café and outside got a terminal transit bus after an hour's wait. He got into it and was drove the ten miles to the port shop. It was the size of a warehouse. He went to the counter, behind it was an Arabic man. He looked at Imoonan then he broke into a smile, jumped over the counter and hugged Imoonan.

"Imoonan my man, how are things, I have not seen you for what? Five years?"

"Yeah, and you're still working here, much action?"

"You know, the governments here, always trying to close us down, then they are influenced by the people who make the billions of dollars here and they back off only to return a year later."

"Yeah, shit, I am looking for an oxygen generator for a class b ship."

"You got the dough, that's an expensive part my friend."

"How much?"

"Well seeing it's my good fiend Imoonan I'll do it ten thousand dollars, you do have dollars don't you?" He produced the envelope and counted out the hundred dollar bills.

"Shit man, you're loaded. I'll order that part, it'll take a couple of hours."

"No bother, I'll hang with you and catch up." They talked about this and that.

"You don't have the Outer Patriots' newspaper? I have not seen this week's."

"Well shit man, that Pete's done it, he made the first psychic party ever in our shitty planet." He looked at the paper. The Arab began talking about the exploits, but Imoonan ignored him, he read. It said,

"In reaction to the city 29's new order Pete and his two friends let off a psychic bomb that heralded the first mass psychic party of our world. The authorities though hunted him down like a criminal and have put him in a controlled detention centre in the north. One friend present at the party said, “It was unreal, I have not seen or heard anything like it, not even on Delta Two…” Delta Two, the place where they have specific festivals dedicated to such parties. Good psychic disc jockeys are revered all over the galaxy…” Imoonan tapped his phone in his hand, if only he could get hold of this Pete.

Chapter 52
Suicidal Happening

Dwight saw a nurse walking over to him with a syringe, he struggled in the straps but could not avoid it. The nurse walked away, Saul said a word of thanks and left the room. The two heavies started to chat to each other.

"What have they done with me?" The heavies stopped the talk, looked at him and then continued their conversation, they ignored any more of Dwight's pleas.

Dwight felt funny, it was like there was a cool wind blowing through his brain. He watched the heavies, that was strange, they seemed to be wearing a tartan that he had not noticed before, and there was a queer smell of cinnamon. Saul re-entered the room. He walked straight up to Dwight and peered at his eyes.

"Yep, it's taking effect, the pupils are fully dilated, where is she?" Someone replied in a slow voice,

"Here I am." Then, "Welcome, Doctor." The room's paint seemed to be running and as he looked at the floor it was covered in green ants. Then,

"We'll do the work, you don't mind if I stay?"

"Of course you can, but he must only hear my voice. Okay?"

"Yes."

"Hello Dwight, my name is Doctor Lavery, today we will be spending some time together. Now I want you to relax, it will all be all right, now look at the little finger of my hand and watch it go from side to side, yes that's it, keep focused on it."

Dwight felt his head swaying, the finger had turned blue and he could hear seagulls. Soon the voice drifted away and it was in his subconscious. He looked around, he was in the smoking room, how did he get here? Oh well, he was away from that Saul and the heavies now. He chilled and began to watch Countdown, he was terrible at the game, he'd just got a four letter word when Pete walked in and sat beside him.

"Hello Pete, still to beat my record of six letters." They began to smoke. Pete began to talk.

"So you know Voodoo man, I killed him, he wanted to be more powerful than me, I tricked him into helping me because of the disturbance, and Joe Bob he is a demon, he let Nile into the world." Dwight looked at Pete, Pete looked back at Dwight, his mind was telling him that this Pete he thought was good was really a bad person. Pete then pulled out a bloody knife and cleaned it on his shirt. Dwight had to tell people about this, the world depended on it, he began to fear Pete and Joe Bob. Why had he been so nice to them? They'd ridiculed him.

"You're so fucking stupid" Pete said to him, then Pete got up and left the room. He felt tired, he went to his room and went for a nap. As he slept he forgot all about the trip to the detention centre. It had been a mistake, after all it had been a very distressing dream.

"And that's that" said Dr Lavery, "Take him home and put him in bed."

When he woke up it was morning. There was a knock at his door, it was Padraic. He'd let him in last night and was told that he was to act like nothing had happened.

"Hello sleepy head." Dwight woke up, he was fine then he remembered Pete, that guy was bad. He shivered at the terror of what he'd learnt in the smoking room. Ryan bumped into him. Dogmatically he said,

"It was a mistake," and walked on.

"Did you see Pete?"

"Yeah he's evil, he killed Voodoo man, and Joe Bob's a demon."

"Are you sure?"

"Yes, Pete is evil and he killed his friend after he helped him with the music." And Dwight walked downstairs. Danny walked passed but gave him a good look, Dwight did not have the same friendly dozy expression, he just looked messed with. Danny went on upstairs. Dwight set about making a brunch, he just did not think of the centre again. Then when he'd finished a slice of toast the doorbell went.

Padraic escorted some people in. It was Oliver and Iris. Padraic pointed Dwight out.

"Hello, we are people from the authorities, we hear you know all about Pete and we want to warn our city 29's citizens, would you come with us?" Dwight did not say anything, he just walked towards them and they guided him to the car, passed Ryan who thought this was getting too bizarre. He called after him,

"They've messed with your head." Padraic put his hand on Ryan's shoulder,

"Leave him, it's all for the good." Ryan shrugged the hand

away and stormed off.

In the car Dwight was dazed. Iris felt a bit guilty but Oliver was glad that things were moving. Once Dwight made his announcement that would be the downfall of Pete and his games.

They arrived at a television studio, and although Dwight would generally have been excited the previous night had dulled him irrevocably. They sat him down. In the room were a camera man and a sound man with a boom. One of Nicola's friends was directing the activities. A prompt screen was place in front for Dwight to read.

"Okay, everyone in their places, good, 3, 2, 1 and action." Then there was quiet, in a slurred mumble Dwight spoke,

"I am here to testify to a murder, (he mentioned Voodoo man's name) and it was committed by Pete. Pete is a Satanist and had used the victim to accomplish a grievous act of black magic that resulted in death." A photo of Pete appeared.

"With my witness the authorities are seeking him and advise the public not to approach him but to phone 999." A photo of Joe Bob was also shown.

"This is his accomplice, known to be dim-witted and under Pete's control. He should also be avoided and if seen the police should also be notified."

"That's a wrap, get it ready for the evening news."

Oliver took Dwight's arm and guided him to a waiting car and he was driven to a psychiatric unit. That was the last that any of his friends saw of him.

Chapter 53
The First Escape of Pete

Pete sat in the sound proof cell. He had to escape, to reassert his fight back into society. Joe Bob was suffering more and more from lethargy. When Pete waved, he did not wave back, he just looked ahead. Then Voodoo man, he became scared with the incarceration and started to talk to the guards when they brought meals in, saying he was innocent and did not really care about Pete's cause, and that he wanted to talk and did not want to be tortured by Tutu again. But it was to no avail.

Again Pete was gassed and brought to the room and strapped to the chair and had an acupuncture needle in his neck. He awoke and there was a television screen in front of him. It was the evening news and the newsreader was saying they had an important announcement. Dwight suddenly appeared. Pete was shocked, he'd never seen anyone he knew on the television, but that was countered by what he said about Pete, how many people would be fooled?

Saul patted Pete on the head,

"See your friend, Dwight's on the TV, eh, ha ha. Talking about you. Ha, ha."

Pete was hauled away. Saul laughed even harder. They had brainwashed Dwight, it was like a show trial that the Soviets had done to their enemies of the state. This was terrible. Pete had to get out, it was getting too much to sort out, he was locked up, away from the life he'd grown to like and had built, now he could not reclaim it.

They brought him back to the cell. Joe Bob looked at Pete and caught his gaze. How could this be? Joe Bob was talking through the glass.

"He had been open all this time" Pete thought as Joe Bob talked to his mind.

"I'll get you out. But you are on your own."

"You won't come?"

"No, life will never take me back, society's gone to shit. I'll stay here for now." Pete glanced away and he noticed the heavies. They talked and kept looking over to the prisoners. Then one of them fell to the ground. The other went rigid and walked over. Like a robot he opened Pete's door.

"What about Voodoo man?"

"So be it." and Voodoo man's door too was opened. The guard was in a deep trance and was acting like a zombie in Joe Bob's control. Pete handcuffed each of them, although he did not lock them in the cells. The two escaped, and walked down a corridor that led them to the stairs that went up to the ground level.

"Beware, step into the office beside you." It was Saul nearby, Joe Bob seemed to be right with them. Saul was saying,

"The plan has all come together, we are back, next the other cities." Saul walked past. Pete opened the door and the prisoners with Joe Bob walked past the stuck up woman in reception who was using a computer. She did not notice them, she was day dreaming about a full promotion in the new state.

"You are free" said Joe Bob. "Go to the public car park at the west edge of the installation. Good bye, I will deal with them, they won't catch you, do not look back."

The two of them were still in their orange jail suits and the car park was about a hundred yards away. They darted about, hiding behind cars and around corners from the various military personnel going about their business. It began to drizzle and then rain heavily; this helped their cause as people ran inside. They made it and there waiting for them was the Professor! Riskily they did not look around to check they would be seen. As an example of Joe Bob's cunning the car park was away from any high buildings from which people might have seen them.

The Professor was equally surprised. Voodoo man jumped in and was crying,

"You came for me Dad, you came." Pete also got in and they both changed out of their orange suits into jeans and jumpers that had been brought along.

"Cheers, Joe Bob again" Pete thought, referring to how the Professor knew to bring a change of clothes for the journey.

"Now get into the car boot, boys." They got in the boot, it being an estate car. It was most uncomfortable and they were on top of each other. As they sped off from the military installation round corners Pete badly bruised his knees. Then the boot was opened.

"Thought those guards would be tough nuts, but they seemed withdrawn and just waved me past after I showed the ID. You Pete must come in and wash, shave and eat. Please." Voodoo man and his father stood together, happy being reunited they both felt blessed by the new father son relationship that had suffered so in the past, what with the Professor's work and the son's delinquency.

"Might I use the phone?" Pete asked.

"Yeah, but you know the score? You were on the television."

"Yeah that was sick, the boy used to live in the same hostel, it was shown to me by the bigwig Saul, he thought it most amusing, bastard."

"Here's the phone." Pete was handed a cordless phone, he dialled the only number he could think of - Jackie's.

"Hello?" said Leo. He found the phone a distraction, those pricks had seized back their power so ruthlessly. He and Jackie's group were in conference.

"Who is it?" he asked.

"It's Pete, put Jackie on." Pete heard an expletive and the phone crash to the floor. Then he heard Leo tell her, then he heard her scream,

"It can't be, it's those Elders trying to trick or incriminate us, be quiet, I'll deal with it." But in her heart she knew it was Pete, it just seemed right.

"Hello." she said warily.

"Pick me up, I am in the north at..." He gave the address. "Are you on your way?" The wind had been knocked out of her, it took her a moment.

"Did you escape? The last I heard…"

"I'll tell you when you pick me up." She hung up and told the others she was "going to pick up Pete!" Everyone in the house was ecstatic, this was the first positive news the group had heard in days since Pete had been picked up. She was tempted to go over the speed limit but decided that that might be risky. Her theory was rewarded as city 29 seemed to be swarming with police cars, and if they'd found out her identity she was sure she'd be harassed.

She pulled into the Professor's driveway and once again Pete got into a car boot. But he did thank his host the Professor for the rescue, and prayed for them.

"Bless you" were the last words Pete said to Voodoo man and his dad.

It seemed there had been divine intervention. There had been the secretary who was at her computer, various workers in the installation and the guards - all let Pete go, then there had been a technical fault with the intelligence people's system for bugging phones, it had all been great for the cause. And now Pete travelled across town amidst a heavy security presence. The word was out, Pete had escaped, but as far as the public were concerned the television had said he was at large anyway. To top it off half the city wanted to help him, only the gullible, brainless people believed Pete was in a Satanic cult, some of them were on the organization's side. Most cared deeply for the rebel. The power the organization had lost would not recover.

Pete looked up at Jackie as she opened the boot. She checked they were not being watched from the neighbouring houses or from the air and stood aside. Pete got out and followed her inside. They went into the lounge. There were cheers and shouts of joy. Pete walked into the middle and took a bow. Several ghosts also made their presence known. There was Wolfie, Pete's oldest friend, there was the Priest who was giggling at how dreamlike and fantastic Pete's recent time had been, and then there was Mocto. In his mind's eye he could also see Kelsang and Alex waving; they floated away happily.

Chapter 54
The Second Escape of Pete

And so the meeting of meetings began. More ghosts drifted in to see.

"The only reason I am here is for the super human exploits of my friend Joe Bob, and I pray his spirit is greatly rewarded, he sacrificed himself so the two of us could leave. And when people see that Voodoo man is alive things will fall away. Trust me. But alas I have no place in this world, I am too big for its boots so to say, I am a loner who hates the fame of his good deeds. What to do?"

The group calmed down. Pete continued.

"You lot, people like you will be the future rulers, it starts today, people shall follow you with jubilation. But what have I to do? I should keep quiet and…"

"I have a solution." said an odd voice to Pete. The others watched him talk to an invisible friend, still feeling glee.

"Okay." said Pete. "Might I use your phone, dear?" he asked Jackie.

"Here use mine, it should be okay" said Julius.

"Thank you. Be back in a minute."

Imoonan was still at the port, he'd fitted the oxygen generator but was hanging out with the Arab warehouse worker. He had pulled out some alien porn and they were having a laugh. His phone rang.

"Probably my bitch sister calling back." But he did not recognize the caller ID. "Hello, Imoonan, galactic trader, what's happening?"

"Ah, I got your number from a mutual friend. My name's Pete, I am told you know of me, would you mind me hitching a lift for a while?"

"Well shit yeah, where are you?"

"City 29, you know it?"

"Not really, but I have an electronic map on my ship. Do you know of any large motorways?"

"Yeah, there's one in the north."

"Okay at 4 am it should be deserted. Bring a flash light and shine it into the sky at that motorway at that time." They both hung up. Imooman turned to the Arab.

"You won't believe it..." the famous Pete calling completely blew both of their minds.

Pete turned to Jackie and the other three.

"Em well looks like I've got my ticket out of here." Mary raised an eyebrow. She suspected something suspicious or underhand.

"Where you going?" asked Leo, he was thinking Pete would run off to Africa.

"Outer space is where I shall go." The room was immediately quiet.

"That's silly, how could you? We need you here." said Jackie.

"What if things don't happen as you say?" went on Jackie.

"I can't be worried, I am going on. I'd like to spend my last hours with you lot in a happy way. I would love you all to come with me to a motorway where I will be picked up at 4am. Let's enjoy the last few hours."

"I am with you Pete." It was Julius.

"It sounds fun and if you are looked after with everyday needs and a new life I envy you." But Julius was sad.

"Right on then" called Pete.

Jackie broke out some cheap champagne and holding her tongue they drank to the future.

"To Pete! To the renegades! To the city! To Joe Bob!" To say Pete was excited was an understatement. He walked up and down. He wanted to go to the motorway now and it was only eleven, then it was midnight, he could not contain himself. Jackie gave him a bag with a bottle of mouthwash, deodorant and a 50 gram pouch of shag tobacco. There were some papers too.

Leo called a Chinese take away. Pete did not know what to get so they ordered the banquet for six with a free bottle of wine. It arrived and the driver asked,

"What's the big party?" He tried to peer through the door way and he got a glimpse of Pete.

"Good God, it's Pete, don't worry I won't tell, good God." And he left. They ate the Chinese and drank the wine. They turned on the television news.

"It turns out that (Voodoo man) was not murdered, he and his father have appeared at our station and in an interview they have revealed mass injustice, but what everyone is asking is - where is

Pete?" It went on. Pete laughed at the fame.

"Well he'll be nowhere in an hour" Jackie quipped.

The time came and they got into a car, no need to hide. Leo drove, Jackie rode shotgun and Pete sat in the middle with Mary and Julius on either side. There was the odd taxi on the road, but that was all, they passed the installation and something was happening there, at this late hour there was a lot of activity. Pete wondered.

Then came the motorway. It had two lanes on each side. They pulled onto the hard shoulder and Pete got out, his legs like jelly. Jackie held his hand. Leo had a torch in his glove box and handed it to Pete. Pete shone it up at the stars. One of them moved, one of the stars moved, it hurtled down from the sky and was about two buses in length, it circled them and then it landed. It had none of the grace of the flying saucers or UFOs seen on television. It crashed down and then thrusters were activated, gently landing it on the ground.

Pete ran towards it and a ramp came down the back of the craft and out popped Imooman. He waved, he was happy, him and Pete were going to make it. They looked at each other for the first time. Imoonan's clothes were from the sixties and Pete's were worn and second hand. The first thing they'd have to do is get some new threads. Great. Pete clambered up the ramp and he took a last look at his friends who stared at this situation with amazement. Up came the ramp and Pete followed Imoonan to the cockpit. It had big front and side windows.

"Hold on my new friend, put the belt on and relax, we are going to have great times." Since the craft had landed several cars had stopped in their tracks and the passengers were on the road watching. One was screaming down a mobile phone. Another was filming it.

The craft only needed another hundred yards to take off, but for the craic he kept to this runway for as long as he could. Flames came out the back, then they were in the air, they looked down on the city then they were in the stratosphere and then they were light years away down the nearest wormhole.

The next week's Outer Patriots paper read,

"PETE LEAVES EARTH IN A BLAZE OF GLORY. CAN BE SEEN NOW AS MONTHLY RESIDENT OF DELTA TWO PARTY."

God looked down on Pete. It was unusual for one to have such impact on many. He had done what was right; he had not been quiet and that was not a sin, he was just a humble schizophrenic, God reflected.

Epilogue

As having the diagnosis of 'schizophrenia' I have experienced most of the things in this book (apart from interstellar travel, maybe in the future) yet I made up the story so as to make things interesting, whether they happened in reality is irrelevant. Pete Brown 6th March 2010.

A Final Poem

Beautiful people are like a light that can't be seen in a blue sky,
They say I'll never amount to anything
I prefer a brown sky.